Taekwondo—Ancient Wisdom for the Modern Warrior

Taekwondo

Ancient Wisdom for the Modern Warrior

Doug Cook

YMAA Publication Center
Boston, Mass. USA

YMAA Publication Center
Main Office
   4354 Washington Street
   Boston, Massachusetts, 02131
   1-800-669-8892 • www.ymaa.com • ymaa@aol.com

POD1108

ISBN:1-886969-93-0

Publisher's Cataloging in Publication
(Prepared by Quality Books Inc.)

Cook, Doug.
   Taekwondo : ancient wisdom for the modern warrior /
Doug Cook. — 1st ed.
   p. cm.
   Includes bibliographical references and index.
   ISBN 1-886969-93-0

   1. Tae kwon do. I. Title.
GV1114.9.C66   796.815'3
                              QBI01-201111

Cover design by Richard Rossiter
Edited by David Ganulan

The author wishes to assure the reader that the use of the personal pronouns
"he" or "she" do not imply the exclusion of any person.

Printed in USA.

This book is dedicated to my wife, Patricia and my daughters, Kristin Lee and Erin Elizabeth, for allowing me the time, that most precious commodity, to practice my passion.

To whatever Energy governs us,

Bless Them

Table of Contents

Foreword

Following many years of diligence and hard work on the part of the World Taekwondo Federation under the direction of Dr. Un Yong Kim, taekwondo has finally gained recognition as a full-medal Olympic sport. This is a major accomplishment considering the high standards set by the International Olympic Committee. As a native Korean, I am particularly proud of this achievement since it characterizes the true nature of the taekwondo spirit. However, it is important to recall that first and foremost taekwondo is a uniquely Korean martial art, as well as a world sport, with roots that date back to antiquity. It is rich in tradition and espouses a philosophy that if approached with sincerity has the potential of enriching the practitioner's life in a variety of ways.

Primarily, taekwondo remains an effective means of self-defense. From the days of the Hwarang warriors of ancient Silla to the present it has consistently demonstrated its defensive value on the field of battle. Aside from its dynamic kicking techniques the art features a complete palette of hand strikes, arm locks and sweeps capable of disabling any assailant. In an effort to instill courage, the taekwondoist drills repeatedly in a series of controlled sparring techniques that strives to eliminate the fear associated with a physical confrontation. Moreover, through the application of the traditional forms, or poom-se, practitioners learn to defend themselves against opponents attacking from various directions thus cultivating agility, focus and strength. In addition, taekwondo has the ability to challenge the mind while nurturing the spirit through a ritual of disciplined practice; perseverance and patience are inculcated as the student moves through the ranks and develops advanced skills.

With the above in mind, it is essential, therefore, that we as martial artists look beyond the modern, competitive aspects of taekwondo in an effort to uncover the treasures that await through a holistic program of comprehensive training. In the past this has proven difficult at best given the scarcity of written material relating to the moral and philosophical components of the martial arts. Having personally authored several books on the subject, I have endeavored to map out the physical techniques of taekwondo in conjunction with their philosophical principles. Both students and colleagues alike have responded well to my work by finding great value in its pages. Consequently, it now gives me great pleasure to look on as one of my students assumes the literary mantle in an effort to forge yet another link in the great chain of knowledge as it relates to taekwondo.

It is clear to me that Mr. Cook is very much devoted to the martial arts through his treatment of the material in this book. Rather then address the physical techniques of the art in a "how to" fashion, as so many have done before, he has chosen instead to juxtapose advanced concepts of taekwondo in parallel with a blueprint for their application in daily life. While reading his work, I have often reflected upon a question many people have inquired about: whether I have ever needed to use my defensive skills in a realistic setting. My reply is that I rely on my knowledge by interacting on a social level with people on a daily basis. Likewise, by embracing the lessons in this book, the martial artist will learn to apply their skill each and everyday in a benign and beneficial manner. The chapters relating to meditation, ki development and personal defense are particularly useful in propagating a greater sense of well being, while the historical sections will animate a past wrapped in conflict and valor.

Furthermore, as a certified black belt instructor Mr. Cook speaks with authority and conviction in describing the many facets of the martial arts. The experience he has gained over the years in establishing his school, the Chosun Taekwondo Academy, has added to his credibility both as a martial artist and a teacher. Truly, if one can teach a technique effectively, they can claim it as their own.

In a world where commercialism prevails, the practice of taekwondo is often misused as a vehicle for self-aggrandizement. Mr. Cook, while maintaining a successful environment in his school, has instead chosen to take the high road by providing his students with a curriculum steeped in tradition. His work here only serves to fortify his elevated approach to an art replete with virtue and wisdom. It is my sincere hope that this volume will act as a global reference guide for generations of taekwondo students to embrace, now and in the future.

Grand Master Richard Chun
9th Dan Black Belt
United States Taekwondo Association

Preface

In my search for knowledge concerning the philosophical and traditional aspects of the martial arts, I have come across a wealth of printed material focusing on various techniques and theory, but very little regarding the practical application of our discipline in living daily life. This void is further compounded when a practitioner enters the martial arts at an advanced age. Many mature students to whom I've spoken share my desire to find documentation to help them find a way to incorporate dojang practices into daily activities. I recall reading a book during an early phase of my training that did address these issues. The emotions it elicited were heart warming to say the least, and fortified my resolve and commitment to the martial arts even further. It was comforting to know that I was not alone in pursuing an endeavor that many would consider a long and difficult road. Taekwondo, my discipline of choice, is built on a foundation of foot and hand techniques that requires the practitioner to develop, among other attributes, strong leg muscles and quick reflexes. Demands placed on the individual by the vigorous training methods can sometimes seem overwhelming, and any sympathy with this frustration is indeed welcome. It is my intention, then, to demonstrate my devotion to the martial arts by attempting to provide a volume worthy of consideration by the serious student.

In today's world, it can be said that a person's moral fiber can be measured by the manner in which they cope with the adversities life sets before them. The way in which the situation is approached and solved, relative to our anxiety, is a function of the ethical stamina we've gained through our life experience. I propose therefore, that diligent training in the martial arts, at whatever age, can prepare the individual to face the aforementioned adversities with the spirit and courage of a modern day warrior.

Acknowledgments

There have been many people and places that have either directly or indirectly influenced this book in some way. It is important to me that I make mention of them here.

Grand Master Richard Chun for his untiring devotion to his many faithful students and to the martial art of taekwondo. Masters Samuel Mizrahi and Pablo Alejandro for their fine instruction and patience. Master Edmund Ciarfella for showing me the path in the first place. The student body of the Chosun Taekwondo Academy for their support. Hoyong Ahn for a great training experience in Korea. David Ripianzi at YMAA for making a dream come true. David Ganulin, my editor and fellow soulmate in the martial arts. Master Jou Tsung Hwa and Loretta Wollering of the Tai Chi Farm in Warwick, NY. Master Yang, Jwing Ming for allowing me to introduce myself. Ms. Johanna Masse of YMAA for answering my emails. John Jordan III and John D. Blomquist, Esq. for reading the drafts. My friends John and Irene Lord, for giving to our dojang. Jose at 1776 Coffee Shop, the Alpine Gourmet Coffee Shop. The Gingerbread House, Cape Hatteras, NC, my tranquil place. My Macintosh IIsi for putting up with my prose on those cold, early mornings. Starbucks coffee. Miss Wiener, my high school English teacher who brought life to my writing. Denny, Dave, and Dawn. Ian Turner Cook, an extraordinary martial artist. And, of course, two of the greatest people I have ever known, my parents, Roy and Joan Cook—the true warriors.

MEMBER:
THE UNITED STATES TAEKWONDO ASS'N.
THE WORLD TAEKWONDO FEDERATION

220 EAST 86TH STREET
NEW YORK, N.Y. 10028
TEL: (212) 772-3700

Richard Chun Taekwondo Center, Inc.

Dear Mr. Cook:

As your Grand Master and President of the United States Taekwondo Association, I congratulate you on the excellence of your book, Warriors of a Different War...Taekwondo Tradition and Philosophy.

Your work speaks with authority based not only on your outstanding qualifications as an instructor, but also with the authority of The Richard Chun Taekwondo Center and the United States Taekwondo Association since your school, The Chosun Taekwondo Academy, is fully accredited by us.

Furthermore, it is obvious to me that your deep devotion to taekwondo has contributed greatly to the value of your book. Those searching for the rich, underlying philosophy that lies within the martial arts, will do well to make this work a welcome addition to their taekwondo library.

I am delighted to write this letter of recommendation and wish you and your taekwondo center every success.

Sincerely yours,

Grand Master Richard Chun
9th dan black belt
President
USTA

Chapter 1

In the Shadow of the Hwarang

You are standing on the Kyongju plain in the ancient kingdom of Silla. The year is 669 A.D. In an effort to secure unification, war has been declared against the neighboring kingdoms of Paekche and Koguryo. All around a battle is raging and sounds of combat fill your ears. Without warning, a soldier on horseback bears down on you. His razor sharp sword gleams brightly in the midday sun. Subordinating all conscious thought, you execute a high, arching crescent kick. The charging animal is startled as the kick makes contact and the horse tumbles to the ground, pinning its rider beneath. Astonished at the potency of this technique, you think back on the endless sessions of intense training this kick took to develop. The gratitude you feel towards your instructor is reflected in a renewed burst of confidence. Safe, at least for the moment, you turn to see from which quarter danger approaches next. Later that night, if a stranger were to eavesdrop on the hushed conversation going on between comrades-in-arms, he might be surprised by the lack of boastful comments regarding those vanquished earlier that day on the field of battle. You and your allies are no ordinary soldiers. You are Hwarang warriors—patriots sworn to live by a strict code of honor.

The dawning of this golden age in Korean martial arts history can be traced back to the mid-seventh century. It was during this period that the tiny

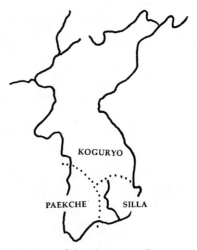

Map of the Three Kingdoms.

1

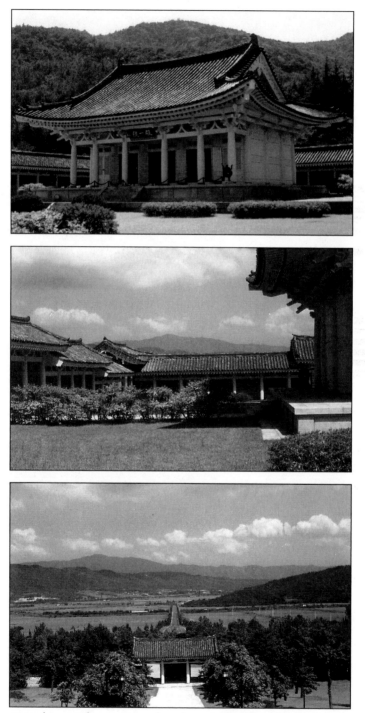

Tong-Il Jeon Palace is situated on the training fields of the Hwarang in what was once the ancient kingdom of Silla.

kingdom of Silla requested aid from neighboring Koguryo in defending its shorelines against the ravages of Japanese pirates. King Gwanggaeto responded by deploying an elite contingent of soldiers numbering 50,000 strong. The warriors brought with them knowledge of *kwonbop,* an advanced system of empty-hand fighting skills. These specialized techniques were, in turn, transmitted to the Sillian army in strict secrecy. In an attempt to increase internal stability, Silla, the smallest and most vulnerable of the three kingdoms, reorganized its government while consolidating its citizenry in answer to the nation's changing needs. This resulted in strong leadership and institutions that reflected the nationalistic spirit of the day. The Hwarang exemplified such an institution.

Founded under King Jin Heung, Hwarang-do or "the way of the flowering manhood," represented a fraternity of Silla's noble elite composed of young people drawn from prestigious families. In addition to being trained in kwonbop and *subahk,* yet another native fighting style, the Hwarang were governed by the Five Codes of Human Conduct. These Five Codes served as a set of moral standards handed down by the Buddhist monk, Wonkwang Popsa, after he was approached by Kwisan and Chuhang, two Hwarang warriors seeking ethical guidance. Among these tenets were those emphasizing loyalty to one's country, the demonstration of respect towards elders, and restraint against the wanton spilling of blood in battle. In an effort to satisfy their spiritual as well as their martial needs, the young warriors

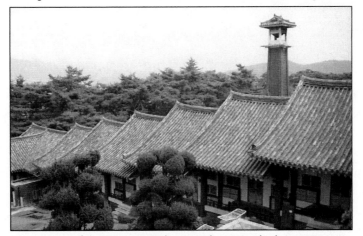

The mission of the Hwarang Educational Institute, built in 1973, is to develop the spirit of the Hwarang in today's Korean students.

of the Hwarang also studied a mixture of music, dance, poetry, and philosophy.

Both Sillian culture and Hwarang-do were heavily influenced by the three major Eastern philosophical paradigms of the day. From the teachings of Confucianism came devotion to state and family, from Buddhism, a heightened sense of commitment to the common good, and from Taoism, belief in the harmonious balance of nature. Originally, divine worship was never intended to play any part in these philosophies-turned-religions. Rather, they were viewed as a path to self-enlightenment or, in the case of Confucianism, a blueprint for ethical behavior. Therefore, by fusing the secret techniques of kwonbop and subahk together with the above principles, Silla's warrior elite was unwittingly setting the stage for a single, cohesive martial philosophy that would endure throughout the centuries. The Korean martial art, taekwondo, as we know it today, is a direct descendant of this rich heritage. Moreover, the ethical standards endemic in its teachings stem from the Hwarang Code of Honor. Shrines and temples still exist that overlook the great expanse of the Kyongju plain, dedicated to the legendary courage and stunning victories of the Hwarang.

Proficiency in the martial arts proved a valuable asset to those living in the seventh century on what would later become the Korean peninsula. But political and geographical considerations have evolved dramatically over the years. Clearly, the martial arts of today are vastly different from those practiced by the Hwarang warriors of the past both in form and spirit. Historically, these styles of empty-hand combat were instituted as a means of unarmed self-defense by those unable to acquire weaponry due to tribal economics or social standing. In all probability, these arts held little philosophical value other than that found in the pride of victory, or the humiliation of defeat.

It was not until the time of Wonkwang Popsa and the Zen patriarch Bodhidharma that a spiritual and ethical tradition began to flourish and permeate the underpinnings of martial philosophy establishing both a virtuous response to threat and a 'way' or 'path' towards superior living. Once imbued in the warrior's structure of thinking, however, it was only a matter of time (albeit centuries) before these elements would cause what was once exclusively battlefield tactics to evolve into the martial arts we are familiar with today. This leads us to the principle question around which this work revolves: What possible benefit can a study of the martial arts, with taekwondo leading the way, offer in a world where we are no longer burdened by the threat of hand-to-hand combat on a daily basis? In order to give this question the proper attention it deserves, we will first examine the history and tradition of taekwondo, determine its definition, and later analyze the physical, psychological, and spiritual promise it holds for the modern day warrior. Let us begin our journey, then, at a most unlikely place—a walk through the fateful shadow cast by the deeds and actions of the noble Hwarang.

Looking back, the period between 660 and 935 A.D. epitomized a true renaissance in Korean societal history. Hwarang-do continued to prosper under Silla's united, highly civilized culture. Maritime trade flourished with Korean ships ruling the waves. The arts and education thrived. State sponsorship of Buddhism resulted in a free exchange of thoughts and ideas between Sillian clerics and their Chinese counterparts. Monasteries were constructed, and a general sense of social consciousness pervaded the country with its rulers effectively leading by example. During this time *taekkyon,* an indigenous martial art featuring circular kicks, enjoyed popular acceptance by the citizenry with demonstrations being performed at festivals and government functions. Students and military personnel were taught the martial arts at specialized training centers located high in the mountains. Much of the prosperity enjoyed during this period has been attributed to the Hwarang who, through indomitable spirit, were responsible for maintaining a strong Korean identity. Even so, by the start of the tenth century, Sillian power began to wane.

It is sometimes difficult to imagine what sociopolitical dynamic would cause a culture as vibrant as Silla's to diminish in stature and eventually dissolve. In truth, the causes were not very distant from those faced by many contemporary societies. Disparity between classes, increasing taxation, and external political pressures all contributed to a shift in government. In what was perhaps the first example of a controlled transfer of power in Asian history, King T'aejo assumed leadership of the self-named

Koryo dynasty, establishing its capital in Sondong. The years between 918 and 1391 A.D. saw many changes in the fabric of Korean society. Although undue taxation was eliminated and a high level of education maintained, the Koryo population suffered many hardships at the hands of the marauding Japanese and Mongol forces, pushing the nation's spirit and defenses to the limit. During this period, gunpowder and other forms of advanced weaponry made an appearance on the field of battle resulting in what was to become a gradual decline in the practical application of the martial arts. Still, the Koryo kings used the native disciplines of subahk and taekkyon as forms of entertainment during state rituals and sporting events. However, the repeated attacks by Japanese pirates and roving bands of Mongols finally took their toll during the latter part of the fourteenth century, destabilizing the government to the point of dissolution.

It was during this period that General Yi-Song Gye stepped in to take control over the disheartened nation. He established the longest surviving government in Korean history. From 1392 to 1910 A.D., the Yi dynasty distinguished itself under the leadership of King Sejong, by creating the Hangul alphabet in 1443—a set of phonetic characters still in use and the pride of the Korean people. Through the use of this alphabet, education evolved even further by allowing the publication of many classical works. Mirrored by a disenchantment with Buddhist beliefs, Confucian ideology had become firmly ensconced in Yi culture as reflected by a strict adherence to literal art rather than those of martial origin. Concerned more with struggles for power, the prevailing leadership allowed the practice of taekkyon and subahk to diminish.

The full effect of this trend would not be felt until 1592 when Japanese forces launched a massive attack against China, using the Korean peninsula, known then as Chosun, as a stepping stone in the process. Essentially defenseless, the population managed not only to survive, but triumph by drawing on the talents of guerrilla units that had been secretly trained in the martial arts at monasteries and estates throughout the region. Out of this conflict came the heroic Admiral Yi, a strategist of unsurpassed proportions whose radical approach to naval warfare played a major role in permitting Chosun to remain independent. Furthermore, the royal government, realizing the error of its ways, began once again to support the martial arts and bolster defenses.

One remaining artifact of this renewal is a volume entitled the *Muyedobo-Tongji,* a text illustrating martial arts techniques fully resembling those practiced today in taekwondo. Nevertheless, the eighteenth and nineteenth centuries found yet another suppression of the martial arts, this time officially sanctioned. Intellectual activities were on the rise, accompanied by the introduction of Christianity. Japan continued its fight for the Korean peninsula, battling first with China and then Russia for dominance over the strategically important nation. Finally, in 1910, after centuries of hostilities, the formal annexation of Korea took place effectively bringing an end to the five hundred-year-old Yi (Chosun) dynasty, and placing the nation under Japanese imperial rule.

During this darkest of times, the Japanese forces attempted to eradicate all vestiges of Korean culture by closing schools, destroying historical documents, and curtailing all practice of the martial arts. Fearing reprisal by their tormentors, many of the original masters of the martial arts went underground after witnessing the persecution and execution of their brethren. Some chose to go into exile, traveling to China or America. Others, forced to serve out the war working in Japan, continued in the martial arts by studying *karatedo.* Fortunately, the spirit of the Korean martial arts was kept alive by rebels training in ancient monasteries and villages scattered throughout the stricken country.

Following the ravages of the Second World War and later the Korean conflict, the nation finally gained its long sought independence from the Japanese and Chinese aggressors. Korean masters returning to their native land once again began to practice the martial arts forbidden by law under the Japanese occupation. In an effort to restore a national identity, the various *kwans,* or martial arts schools, began negotiations in April of 1955 aimed at uniting their styles under a single banner that would eventually come to be known as taekwondo. Since that time, the Asian martial arts have become a combined source of mystery and curiosity in the minds of many Westerners. American military personnel returning from battle-torn Korea brought with them tales describing unarmed fighting arts in sharp contrast to the pugilistic sporting styles familiar to those back home.

As legend had it, masters of diminutive stature would send brawny servicemen flying through the air with a simple twist of the hips. Others, it was claimed, endowed with a secret knowledge of mind over matter, could kill with a single, well-placed blow. Some veterans who wished to continue their training after gaining proficiency in the martial arts overseas, acted as sponsors in obtaining American citizenship for their Asian mentors. Aside from a show of gratitude and respect, this action was undoubtedly motivated by the realization that there were very few teachers in the United States at the time capable of offering quality instruction. Original taekwondo pioneers such as Richard Chun, Henry Cho, and Jhoon Rhee continue to leave their mark on the martial arts community. Consequently, it was not long before schools began to spring up—first on the West Coast and then in major cities across the nation. Even suburbia, no longer immune to what can only be characterized as an explosive growth curve, boasts an abundance of training halls located in the ubiquitous strip malls and shopping centers.

In the distant past, many of the Asian martial arts were considered secret weapons by the family, tribe, or nation by which they were developed. Clearly, this is no longer the case. With differing styles jockeying for legitimacy and the recognition of taekwondo by the International Olympic Committee, what began as a system of self-defense in the 1950's has matured into a $1.5 billion American industry. Although this trend has spurred heated controversy in certain circles given the traditional values associated with the martial arts, one cannot deny the impact it has had on making instruction more accessible to the masses.

This is particularly evident in the case of taekwondo where the flicker of hope that existed in post-war Korea eventually ignited an intense flame of interest in a portion of the general public inclined towards a study of the martial arts. This acceptance was partially driven by the high standardization of various techniques and forms unique to the Korean martial art. Organizations such as the World Taekwondo Federation under the direction of Dr. Un Yong Kim, the United States Taekwondo Association founded by Grand Master Richard Chun, and the International Taekwondo Federation headed by General Choi Hong Hi, have been responsible for blending these techniques into a cohesive curriculum that has made taekwondo the fastest growing martial art in the world today.

Literally translated, taekwondo is defined as 'foot-hand way,' or the art of smashing with hands and feet. These translations, while direct, are incomplete at best since they only hint at the myriad of moral and ethical benefits associated with this noble, Korean discipline. For decades taekwondo has been the perfect vehicle for cultivating inner strength, extraordinary endurance, and an effective arsenal of defensive skills. In its current iteration it can be thought of as a direct reflection of modern society's desire for a ritualized discipline devoid of religious dogma, but complete with both physically and spiritually enhanced sets of ethical principles by which to live. Beyond this, as the reader will soon come to realize, lies a universe filled with intangibles relating to the very essence of the art. For one, taekwondo has a proclivity for transforming even the most cynical man or woman into a spiritually enlightened person displaying a renewed passion for life. This seemingly impossible task is accomplished by constantly reminding the practitioner of their self-worth and unique place in the cosmic scheme of events.

Because we are living in a world of sometimes overwhelming proportions, technology, financial obligations, even the size of the buildings in which we live and work, can result in a feeling of insignificance. Therefore, by shunning conformity in the name of art, taekwondo allows room for personal expression beckoning the student to cultivate self-esteem through individuality. Moreover, taekwondo is an empowering art. It is a holistic method for nurturing internal strength by way of acquired skill. By this standard, the more frequently one trains and becomes proficient in the martial arts, the more one realizes they have less to defend against. Confidence begins to replace fear. Defensive skills become ingrained, resulting in one's ability to walk life's path appreciating its simple pleasures rather than being blinded by its daily perils. Therefore, contemporary taekwondo, taught in a traditional manner, is not merely about physical enhancement (although that will occur naturally over time), but about spiritual fulfillment—the goal of which is to clear a path in preparation for the martial artist to embrace the virtues and rewards life has to offer.

The emotional wars the modern day warrior must face on a daily basis are most likely very different from those fought by the Hwarang. While many of the physical techniques have remained intact, the weaponry and protagonists, being of a starkly dissimilar nature, have radically changed over time requiring an improved suit of armor. This garment must be woven with the threads of self-esteem, the leather of confidence, and the metal of perseverance. Traditional taekwondo, as the reader shall discover, if practiced with diligence and sincerity, is certain to provide the raw materials necessary to construct just such a suit of armor.

CHAPTER 2

A House of Discipline

Every organization has as its focal point, a physical center. For government, it is a capitol. For the various religious denominations it can be a church, temple, or mosque. For taekwondo, this center is called a dojang. In the Korean language, *do* can be defined as "art" or "way." A *dojang,* therefore, is a place of honor where the modern day warrior comes to practice the Way. Literally meaning "gymnasium" or "training hall," a dojang can also be a house of discipline—a solemn location devoid of superfluous frivolity. By stepping onto the mat, the practitioner is crossing the threshold of commonality into a world rich in the superior attributes of life. They are declaring to themselves and those around them that they are prepared to meet the rigorous challenges set forth by a serious study of the martial arts. The training is never easy and requires a great deal of commitment and patience. Expectations run high in this supercharged environment, both on the part of the instructor as well as the student. It is here that the novice, in his infancy, is taught the most fundamental of techniques. It is here also that the mature practitioner accepts the awesome responsibilities that go hand in hand with becoming a black belt.

However, in the same way that a house does not necessarily make a home, a dojang can potentially be a cold and sterile shell; a room surrounded by four square walls if not for the soul that fills it. This soul is personified primarily by the philosophy and traditional values espoused by the master instructor, followed by the enthusiasm and devotion radiated by its students. Furthermore, the distinct elements of physical space, ideology, human form, and spirit, combine to create what many perceive as being the unique flavor associated with a particular school. But just as no two individuals can claim to possess identical souls, so it is that no two schools are truly alike.

The fact that there can be very obvious differences between two schools of the same "style," never fails to raise an eyebrow among newcomers who automatically assume that any practice of the martial arts represents a rigid structure of movements, uniform in style, and unchanged since time immemorial. This impression of inflexibility is understandable given the classical nature of taekwondo, an art with roots that have been handed down from master to disciple over the centuries. Although various worldwide governing bodies regulate the vast majority of techniques found in taekwondo, much of a school's daily curriculum continues to be dictated by the strengths and weaknesses of its master instructor. Typically endowed with years of experience, this human icon single-handedly sets the mood, tempo, and intensity of dojang life. As an example, students will often mirror the proclivities of their masters. If a teacher exhibits a liking towards a certain kicking technique, chances are the student will generally reflect this pronounced ability. Conversely, the master of one dojang may favor the use of vigorous sparring drills during the course of each class, while another might stress martial arts philosophy and meditation instead. Presuming this schism in traditional teaching methods exists, what standards should an interested party go by in selecting an appropriate dojang to meet their individual requirements and goals? What attributes should one look for in a school's instructors? And finally, how does the potential student go about locating a reputable dojang in the first place?

To begin with, the martial arts community appears to be entering an era of professional adolescence. With its popularity waxing, it has become a vehicle for the veteran practitioner to transform his hard-earned skills into a lucrative commercial venture. But as with any burgeoning industry, the possibility of turning a quick profit has encouraged a darkened few to subvert well intentioned, pure at heart individuals through the use of manipulation and other questionable sales tactics. This phenomenon is particularly interesting, considering the foundation of honor on which taekwondo is built. Fortunately, those who wholly embrace the complex process of transmitting quality martial arts skills to their students outnumber these charlatans. One method of measuring these varying degrees of competency and forthrightness is by obtaining the recommendations of a grateful student body.

Metaphorically speaking, it is rare that an individual, suffering some form of ailment, would choose to be treated by an unknown physician. More likely, the person would seek a referral, either from a trusted acquaintance or other qualified source. So it is with taekwondo. On the other hand, taekwondo centers will sometimes advertise in school or community newsletters, and most certainly in local newspapers. Occasionally, flyers extolling the virtues of various schools can be found hanging on bulletin boards in shopping centers. By the same token, telephone directories, especially those in greater metropolitan areas, generally contain multiple listings under the headings of "karate" or "martial arts," identifying schools in the vicinity. Shopping for a dojang by phone should be done on a superficial level only, leaving details to be discussed in person. At any rate, no commitment should be made, either verbal or written, until the perspective student views a class in progress.

By visiting a dojang recommended by a current student or being invited to attend a trial class by a reputable instructor, the novice will have an opportunity to observe the atmosphere, traditions, and teaching methods of the school's instructors first hand. This is clearly the first step in any diligent study of the martial arts. Once there however, there are certain indicators of which the aspiring martial artist should be aware.

Upon entering the dojang, after taking note of the large American and Korean flags that typically decorate the head of the room, the observer should sense an air of anticipation emanating from the students waiting to begin class. This is not a form of nervous energy, but rather a manifestation of *ki,* the internal life force a martial artist must learn to cultivate and project over time. The students are acting in a dignified manner, leaving conversation for later and stretching in preparation for the training that lay ahead. Their uniforms are clean, and of the traditional taekwondo fashion. All the practitioners who planned to attend this class are present, realizing how inconsiderate it would be to arrive late, breaking the concentration of both the instructor and fellow students upon entering the dojang. At this point, the teacher steps onto the mat and the entire class comes politely to attention, bowing in a humble show of respect. All eyes are looking straight ahead, feet are planted firmly together with hands at the sides in anticipation of the master's opening words.

Since our daily lives are generally filled with more than the practice of taekwondo, it is at this point that the students are asked to free their mind of any extraneous thoughts that may hinder the training process through the use of meditation. As we shall see in later chapters, meditation can be used to great advantage by the martial artist both during class as well as in everyday life. The amount of emphasis a school places on the spiritual aspects of taekwondo can be gauged by how this period of meditation is approached. After receiving the command of *Muk Yum* (meditation) from the instructor, the students will kneel briefly with eyes closed in an attempt to clear the mind of all daily affairs. Rituals such as these are commonplace in the martial arts. Depending upon the style or national origin of the discipline, this may include a salute to the flags, mention of the various ethical tenets particular to a school or, in some cases, a form of respect displayed towards the founder of a given art. This done, the class is ready to begin training.

By now, the potential student should have formulated some opinion regarding the level of seriousness the instructor and students attach to their training. The opening ritual sets the tone for the vigorous mental and physical exercises that are to follow and affords the novice an opportunity to experience the dignity and respect so essential in taekwondo. One would seriously need to question a school's devotion to discipline if, during this portion of the class, the students' thoughts appeared to be wandering, or the instructor displayed an inability to inspire self-control.

The study of taekwondo requires homage be paid to the body as a whole, not simply the mind, body, or spirit individually. Consequently, given the previous attention shown towards martial decorum, it becomes the responsibility of the qualified instructor to prepare the student physically prior to a strenuous workout. It is a fact that chances of injury decrease proportionally to the amount of time allotted for stretching and aerobic exercise. Some schools will allow as much as a full half-hour for warm up exercises alone. Attempting to execute high, jumping kicks or effective punches without the appropriate warm-up will

Standard Class Curriculum

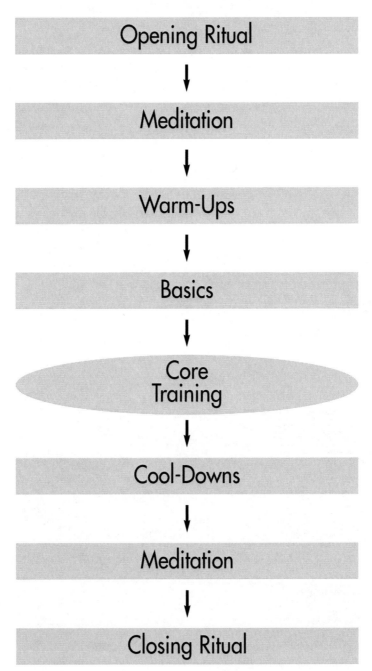

only result in pulled hamstrings or sore shoulders. Many of the stretching exercises unique to taekwondo are similar to those found in dance. It is not uncommon to find the martial artist with legs extended, one perched atop a bar or straining for those few extra inches while seated in a front split.

Since taekwondo is a defensive martial art however, these exercises must also be accompanied by those capable of strengthening arm, leg, and stomach muscles. Jumping jacks, push-ups, and leg raises, in conjunction with weight training and a number of other complex combinations, answer this need. In either case, these routines enhance the overall physical fitness and flexibility of the practitioner, allowing them to lead a stronger, healthier life in general. If this is a primary goal, witnessing a thorough warm-up session as a prelude to a taekwondo class will leave no doubt in the mind of the novice that they are on the right track. A dojang concerned with the total well being of its students will tend to stress this portion of the curriculum. The training that follows the series of warm-up exercises lies at the very core of taekwondo and gives, perhaps, the greatest indication of a school's worth. Clearly, the goal of any reputable dojang is to offer the student a well-rounded and complete education in the martial arts, the depth of which can range anywhere from specialized abilities in women's self-defense tactics to proficiency in Olympic-style competition sparring.

However, any attempt at describing a "typical" taekwondo class would be presumptuous at best considering the variety of

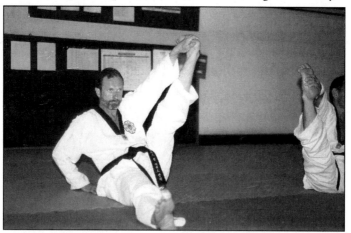

A dojang can be judged on the attention given to warm-ups.

backgrounds and teaching methods employed by the art's various masters. Suffice it to say that taekwondo is not just about fighting as many imagine, but offers the ultimate reward of self-fulfillment achievable through the scientific mix of physical, mental, and spiritual philosophies taught in the dojang. It is essential that the novice observe this segment of the course closely, matching their aspirations with the strengths of the school because this is where the bulk of the strategies and techniques specific to taekwondo are demonstrated. Moreover, how an instructor chooses to translate these concepts into coordinated action will, in large part, determine the long-term compatibility between him and his students.

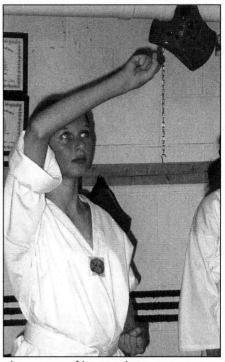

The practice of basic technique is an essential component of the art of taekwondo.

For instance, traits that positively motivate certain individuals may have a negative effect on others. Some taekwondoists thrive in an atmosphere rich in discipline since this aspect may have proven fundamental in their initial attraction to the martial arts. Others however, may flock to a teacher showing signs of a more compassionate nature. Both are acceptable provided the instructor continues to command a level of respect. During this trial period, it is important for the observer not to become discouraged by what they are seeing. Younger students or those with more experience may be performing endurance drills or the dramatic jumping kicks that have become the hallmark of taekwondo. This may result in an overwhelming sense of frustration on the part of the novice. How instructors deal with the awe and innocence of the beginner is still another indicator of a school's worthiness. Occasionally, if it is feasible, some dojangs will segregate students according to belt rank, arranging separate classes for white and yellow belts. This allows the novice to proceed at his or her own pace rather than being driven or intimidated by those further along.

Yet another topic that the future martial artist should consider is one that is presently generating considerable debate in modern taekwondo— that of the distinction between martial art and martial sport. While this issue will be dealt with later on in greater detail, it is worth mentioning here simply because many of today's schools and instructors strongly emphasize this athletically weighted aspect of taekwondo. With the possibility of a competitor gaining international recognition looming in the distance, taekwondo's inclusion as an Olympic sport has become the driving force in attracting a multitude of potential practitioners. This is especially true in the case of young adults and teenagers whose parents see this as an opportunity to have their offspring learn the skills and discipline associated with a highly competitive sport. If this represents the final goal of the aspirant, a dojang should be chosen based on its application of endurance drills, footwork, and overall competitive strategies. A draw unto itself, the sport derivative of taekwondo has acted as the catalyst for much of the unification and growth of the art. While nowhere is it written that one form of training should supplant the other, that the artful and athletic pursuits of taekwondo cannot conceptually coexist, the novice should bear in mind that training for international, national, or even local full-contact competition can be radically different from that found in the traditional approach to martial arts training. Schools featuring or specializing strictly in classes geared towards tournament sparring must, in their instructor's zeal for victory, never loose sight of a classic lesson taught by taekwondo: that the most truculent and elusive opponent one can conquer is oneself.

Realizing that the martial arts of today have been redefined in terms of their originally intended, purely defensive value, there are those who have chosen to join the ranks of the taekwondoist in search of meaningful social interaction with contemporaries sharing similar interests. Enrollment lists are filled with the names of concerned, intelligent men and women who have become jaded and bored with the standard aerobic and exercise programs. These people have turned to taekwondo seeking an alternative method of physical fitness, discipline, and self-awareness. It is surprising how quickly the novice, after only a class or two, begins to experience the passion that is commonly seen in the eyes of the veteran martial artist. The bond this feeling creates between members of a dojang contains an ingredient of camaraderie whose power has the ability of cementing relationships far superior to those found in other facets of society. On a domestic level, dojangs are offering attractive membership rates that cater to the family unit in hopes of introducing the martial arts as a wholesome way to spend quality time together. Parents and siblings interact as equals, sharing the gratification found in working towards a common goal.

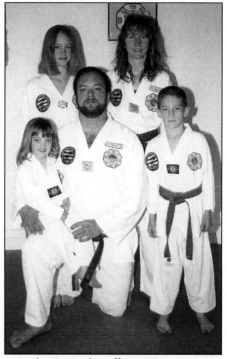

Most dojangs today offer training programs that cater to the whole family.

So far, we have learned how to make contact with a dojang, what to expect from an average class, and what attributes to look for in a school and its instructors. But what of the physical environment of a dojang? What effect does this aspect have on a newcomer's desire to train at a given location? Like the health club or aerobics studio, the novice may gravitate towards a gymnasium that is clean, well lit, and contains modern, well-maintained equipment. Many students are drawn to a dojang by amenities such as the rubberized safety floor, wall mirrors, weight training equipment, kicking targets, and locker rooms with showers. These features lend an

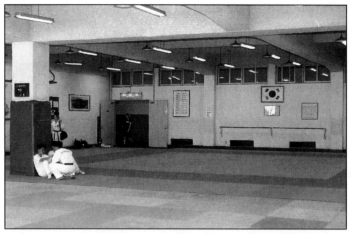

Since there is no set rule dictating the architecture of a dojang, a number of styles exist around the world. This dojang is at the Korean National University of Physical Education in Seoul, Korea.

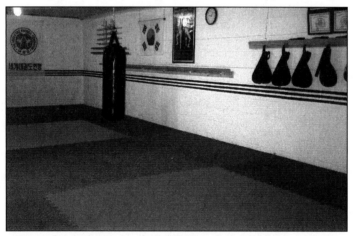

A dojang located in the basement of a New York home.

air of permanence and professionalism to a school and offer a convenience to business people taking classes before work or during their lunch break. But the trophies in the front window and the medals on the wall do not tell the full story behind the image. It is often said that perception is more important than reality. While this may be true in politics or advertising, it is simply not the case in taekwondo. Substance, by all means, takes precedence over form. Once again, we come back to the students, the black belts and upper belts who, viewed as a

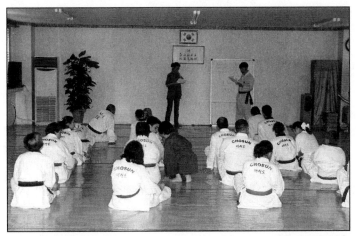

A school in Seoul, Korea emphasizing the cultivation of ki, a vital life force.

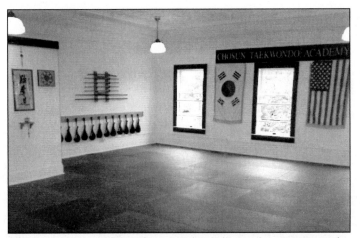

The present home of the Chosun Taekwondo Academy in Warwick, New York.

barometer, epitomize and mirror the instructor's ability to successfully transmit the martial tradition with sincerity and integrity. These dichotomies were twice demonstrated to me in dramatic fashion, both times during a training excursion to Korea, the homeland of taekwondo.

On the first occasion, the benefit of substance over form became abundantly clear inside the doors of Il Shim, a humble dojang located in Yesan, a few hours drive west of Seoul. Translated as "One Heart," Il Shim can be reached by taking a leisurely stroll through the center of town and up the winding back roads dotted with merchants supplying customers with red peppers, garlic, and raw fish. Turning down a side street with the unmistakable scent of kimchee wafting through the air, one finds himself standing before the gates of an unassuming two-story dwelling. Unlike its American counterpart, Il Shim does not boast a neon sign in its front window proclaiming it to be a school of taekwondo. On the contrary, there is no overt mention of its true mission or that of its owner. Once inside, the wooden floor, patched and worn, becomes obvious, lending credence to the dedication invested in the dojang by its founder, Grand Master Bung Hoo Yoo. An eighth dan, this quiet, confident man has trained many students in the art of taekwondo and claims to have graduated as many as seven hundred black belts. Situated in the building's basement, the sparsely decorated walls of Il Shim are adorned only by a small Korean flag and framed photographs of the Grand Master with some of his students turned national champions. Off to one side sits an aged set of weights, while on the other, a room in which children are seated at a long bench completing homework prior to their training. There is wonder in the faces of the youngsters as they stare at us wide-eyed, most never having seen Westerners before. In celebration of our visit, Grand Master Yoo called his students to attention and had them perform the taekwondo *poom-se* or forms he had so painstaking-ly taught them. Resounding with spirit shouts, the dojang came alive as the youthful martial artists moved across the floor, displaying crisp, determined movements. Next, in reciprocity of the honor extended us, our junior students rendered a series of similar forms, much to the delight of the combined audience. The communication passing between the two groups was not limited by the words of the translator, but rather, expanded on by the universal language of the taekwondoist who shares the same techniques with his colleagues in over one hundred countries. Later, seated in a circle of solemn respect, we listened as Grand Master Yoo spoke with subdued pride of his dojang's history and the memories he collected furthering the art of taekwondo.

In a second and separate encounter during the same training expedition, we were honored to visit The Korean National University of Physical Education in Seoul. It is here that the elite

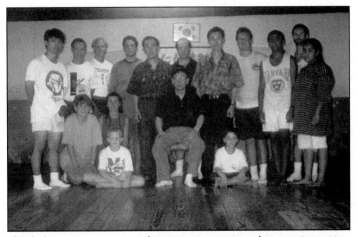

The Il Shim or "One Heart" dojang in Korea. Grand Master Bung Hoo Yoo (seated) maintains his dojang on the ground floor of his home.

of Korea's youth train and reside in hopes of qualifying for the Korean National Team and competing in the Olympics. As our bus pulled into the main entrance, we noticed students strolling around the campus grounds with sparring gear poking out of their gym bags. With a modicum of trepidation, the realization began to sink in that we were about to face some of the world's most capable taekwondo practitioners. Our fears were somewhat assuaged, however, by recalling the thread of mutual respect that runs through the heart of all martial arts training. With this in mind, we entered the locker rooms and changed into our *doboks*. It was with a feeling of deep pride and honor that we came to attention before beginning what was to be the most demanding class we had ever experienced.

Beside our group of fourteen, there were twenty other practitioners from Korea and other countries in the gymnasium-sized dojang. Because the duration of a typical class may range anywhere from three to eight hours, there is a substantial amount of time initially allocated for endurance training. We began class by thoroughly stretching and continued with some aerobic exercises, running, kicking and executing splits while jumping across the floor in various directions. Next came the kicking drills. Using targets, these drills were aimed at increasing our focus and strength while perfecting our combination attacks. Eight lines were formed with the students being divided equally among them. Each line was headed by one of our hosts from the university who held two kicking targets, one in each hand. Moving forward, backward and to the side in rapid succession, the object of this exercise was to focus our kicks wherever our partner placed the target in space. Speed and accuracy were of the essence. Following the drills we were told to line up in size order and were then treated to a period of free fighting with these superb Korean martial artists. Our earlier fears evaporated in the heat of the moment, for while our sparring partners were blindingly fast and proficient due to their intense training, it quickly became apparent that they realized we came to Korea to learn from them and not simply to compete. It is interesting to note that a debate continues regarding the issue of whether American martial artists are equipped with the stamina and discipline to endure the rigorous teaching methods used in training their Korean counterparts. In truth, during our training with the Korean Taekwondo Team, we were required to expend considerably more energy than we were normally accustomed to. But, by virtue of the vigorous training methods we had become accustomed to back home, we managed to perform well.

It is difficult to describe the inherent difference in attitude between American and Korean practitioners and their dojangs. As a result of their ancient heritage and national pride, the Korean martial artist takes his training quite seriously. This was a quality we detected in all the Korean taekwondoists we came in contact with during our travels. Beneath the surface, however, we were collectively pleased to discover that we all spoke a common language, a language of kicks, blocks, and a love of taekwondo. These interactions cause one to conclude that it is not the material wealth of a dojang that marks its effectiveness, but the skills and compassion inherent in its master and instructors that creates a distinction.

As we can see, whether in Korea or America, discipline in both thought and action is a concept that clearly needs to be learned and cultivated since it is not necessarily an attribute that comes naturally. Discipline dictates the manner in which a person approaches matters of finance, labor, nutrition, and most importantly, the art of taekwondo. Dojangs have the ability to inculcate this elusive quality by means of the demands placed on the practitioner in embracing the martial arts. For this very reason, by seeking the Way in such a center, the modern warrior can expect to become better equipped in dealing with the issue of complacency. By drawing strength from the dojang, in conjunction with the application of the code of honor that lies at the very soul of taekwondo, the sincere practitioner will rapidly come to see the value in a disciplined way of life.

CHAPTER 3
A Code of Honor

Honor can be defined as a sense of what is right, just and true; a dignified respect for character, springing from principle or moral rectitude. From the ubiquitous bow of respect practiced from the moment a student enters the dojang to the deference afforded a grand master, honor is clearly an integral part of the martial arts. However, as one can imagine, the concept of honor, especially as it is applied to the art of taekwondo, did not originate in modern times. Rather, it stems from a history rich in martial virtue.

For as long as one can remember, most of the world's leading martial ways, regardless of origin, have clearly encouraged the cultivation of a refined moral character. Although fundamental differences exist between styles, the end result is ideally the same—holistically enlightened individuals, adroit in the ways of self-defense, living by an implied code of honor that has been developed over the course of history by cultural necessity. How did this union between the martial arts (clearly a pursuit resonant with aggressive overtones) and morality come about? In order to answer this question we must look not only to ancient Korea, but also to China—a country rich in martial arts history. There, in the early sixth century, the amalgam between fighting art, honor and religion begins to materialize when we examine the life of the Zen Buddhist patriarch, Bodhidharma, third son of the Brahman Indian king, Sagandha.

Early references are made to Bodhidharma's association with a warrior caste during his youth known as the Kshatriya. It was through this association that he was schooled in the empty-hand fighting art of *vajramushti*. It is conjectured that Bodhidharma traveled to Hunan Province in northern China eventually finding his way to the fabled Shaolin Temple. Upon his arrival, Bodhidharma discovered that the clerics inhabiting the monastery were incapable of practicing advanced meditation techniques due to their weakened state of mind and body. Frustrated with his findings, Bodhidharma sequestered himself in a cave for a period of nine years meditating and authoring two books in the process. It is said that Bodhidharma suffered this self-imposed exile while waiting for a worthy disciple to appear, one whom he felt was deserving of his teachings. When one finally did arrive in the tenth year, the potential candidate attempted to prove his devotion by severing his arm off in order to demonstrate his appreciation for the difference between internal desires and external, material needs. As a result, the Shaolin monks to this day raise one hand when bowing to Buddha as a show of respect to their predecessor. At that point, no doubt drawing on his past experience, Bodhidharma returned to the temple and initiated a program of exercise drills that came to be known as *Shih Pa Lo Han Sho* or "The Eighteen Hands of Lo-Han." Considering Bohidharma's Zen background, these exercises were, in all likelihood, initially intended as a non-violent form of discipline, but may well be credited with spawning many of the Chinese fighting styles we are familiar with today, the most noteworthy being *gongfu*. These techniques were imparted with the hope of strengthening the monk's ability to concentrate dur-

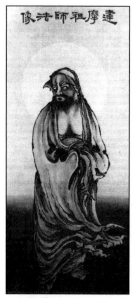

Bodhidharma (Da Mo)

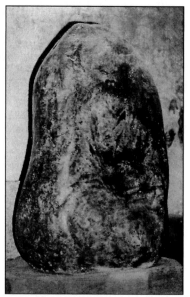

Rock with Bodhidharma's image found at the place where he meditated.

ing their meditation while preserving the spiritual harmony required in monastic life. Furthermore, since their religious background forbade the use of weapons, teaching the Shaolin monks how to defend themselves against wild animals and marauding bandits through the use of empty-hand techniques during their travels, came as a secondary benefit. It is also said that Bodhidharma was responsible for showing the clerics methods to cultivate the vital life force, known as *ki,* in the form of Da Mo's *Wei Dan* (Bodhidharma's Internal Elixir). Aimed at concentrating this internal energy within a specific part of the human anatomy, these exercises are said to be the precursor to modern day *qigong.*

Even at this early developmental stage, we begin to see a connection between the physical, spiritual, and ethical dimensions of the martial arts in relationship to Eastern religion. But what of the conceptual definition of honor as it equates to combat? When we think of honor in battle, two warrior sects from distant parts of the world quickly come to mind: King Arthur's Knights of the Round Table with their renowned Code of Chivalry, and the Japanese samurai whose behavior and philosophy was greatly influenced by the doctrine of *Bushido.* The term "Bushido" contains three distinct components: *Bu,* meaning martial arts, *shi* meaning warrior, and *do* often translated as "the way" or "the path." Taken together, Bushido then can be defined as, "the way of the samurai," or "the way of the warrior." Taisen Deshimaru Roshi, a Japanese Zen Buddhist master born of a samurai family, reveals that Bushido consists of seven basic principles:

> *Gi: The right decisions taken with equanimity, the right attitude, the truth. When we must die, we must die, rectitude.*
>
> *Yu: Bravery tinged with heroism.*
>
> *Jin: Universal love, benevolence toward mankind, compassion.*
>
> *Rei: Right action, courtesy.*
>
> *Makoto: Utter sincerity, truthfulness.*
>
> *Melyo: Honor and glory.*
>
> *Chugo: Devotion, loyalty.*

Furthermore, Deshimaru Roshi goes on to point out the profound effect Shintoism and Buddhism, both Eastern religions, have had on Bushido. The elements of these philosophies found in the samurai code of honor include:

- *Pacification of emotions*

- *Tranquil compliance with the inevitable*

- *Self-control in the face of any event*

- *A more intimate exploration of death than of life*

- *Pure poverty*

Established between the twelfth and seventeenth centuries as a guide for social and ethical behavior, these qualities dovetailed with the daily existence of the samurai warrior who was patently willing to sacrifice his life for that of his master at a moment's notice. Possessing the fortitude and philosophical depth it took to courageously face life and death with equal resolve by virtue of this code became an essential prerequisite for these early martial artists.

In the case of taekwondo, however, much of this virtuous thought in response to military and social necessities can be traced to the moral actions surrounding the select members of the Hwarang. As much as six hundred years prior to the development of Bushido, we find these celebrated warriors of ancient Silla practicing their own unique code of honor under the banner of Hwarang-do. The Hwarang, as we have seen, were an elite group of young patriotic nobles schooled in the ways of contemporary art, philosophy, and martial discipline in temples located high in the distant mountains of ancient Korea. From this group were chosen many of the tiny kingdom's illustrious kings, government officials, and formidable military leaders. Attainment of such esteemed station did not come easy and was made possible only through the practice of the three scholarships: royal tutor, instructor and minister, and the six ways of service: holy minister, good minister, loyal minister, wise minister, virtuous minister and honest minister. But it was during the thirtieth year of King

Chin-Hung's rule in the early seventh century, that a most profound event took place that would eventually have a significant effect on traditional taekwondo. Approached by the two young Hwarang warriors Kwisan and Chuhang, the Buddhist monk Wonkwang Popsa, while residing at Kusil temple on Mount Unman, handed down the five commandments for exemplary living based on Confucian and Buddhist doctrine. These principles, known as the *Sesok Ogye,* became the Code of the Hwarang and are paraphrased and taught today under the heading of The Student Creed of Taekwondo.

Sesok Ogye

(Code of the Hwarang)

Loyalty to the King

Obedience to Parents

Trust among Friends

Never retreat in Battle

Justice in Killing

In addition to these five directives were a set of nine moral virtues the combination of which resulted in a comprehensive set of ethical standards for exemplary living. These principles, as we shall see in later chapters, were indeed taken seriously by the Hwarang as an interpretation of the warrior way. They are portrayed in ancient chronicles memorializing great acts of valor in time of war.

Nine Moral Virtues

Humility	*Courtesy*	*Wisdom*
Justice	*Trust*	*Goodness*
Virtue	*Loyalty*	*Courage*

Still, while it is possible to understand how a soldier on an ancient field of battle would rely on metaphysical beliefs and ethical principles to make some sense of his surroundings and almost certain demise, how do we weigh the concerns of the modern day warrior living in a vastly revised geopolitical environment? Today's warrior is not the trained, professional soldier, but the average man or woman who has turned to the martial arts in search of spiritual enlightenment as well as physical and mental development. This individual may be wondering if honor continues to hold the same meaning today as it did fourteen centuries ago and if so to what extent? Furthermore, how do we transpose the martial concept of honor into a useful quality to be practiced today in our own daily life?

Regardless of the fact that the majority of us will never be called upon to prove our skills in the heat of battle, life and the obstacles it presents offer just cause to seek out and develop an elevated set of noble principles.

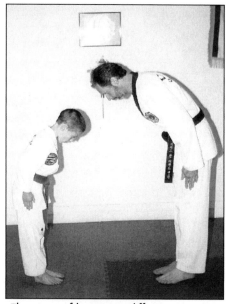

The virtue of honor is indifferent to age or belt rank. An instructor and young student bow to one another.

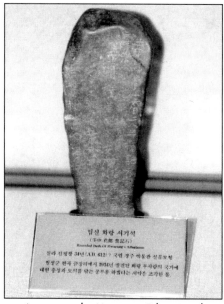

A stone at the Hwarang Educational Institute in Korea inscribed with the Hwarang Oath of Allegiance.

Consequently, the lens of ethical behavior truly magnifies the worthiness of martial arts training since the way we deal with life's adversities is directly proportional to the depth of our ethical standards.

For example, today in our own society, just as in the past, the importance of nurturing an overriding code of moral behavior becomes evident when the physical capabilities one attributes to the martial arts are taken into account. In his book, *Living the Martial Way*, Forrest E. Morgan states "Only honor separates the thugs from the warriors." Once endowed with the deadly fighting skills unique to the martial arts, soldiers such as the samurai and the Hwarang could easily have turned their knowledge to sinister means thus negating the true intentions of their masters and superiors. Likewise, practitioners of the arts today are no more immune to these dangers than their predecessors. In reality, historical precedent exists that documents periods where fighters skilled in the martial arts have risen up against society. Following the destruction of the Shaolin temple by Manchu forces in 1570, many of the surviving monks went underground hoping to sustain their art. In response to government suppression, however, secret societies known as the Triads arose. One such group, the White Lotus Society, was highly successful in their quest for superiority by utilizing martial arts skills against their enemies. Later, in the throes of the bloody Boxer Rebellion during the summer of 1900, Chinese fighters again used martial arts techniques in an attempt to expel invading European troops from Beijing. Developments of this sort were, however, not unique to China. In the aftermath of the Korean conflict, for example, it is rumored that some of the more aggressive kwans, or martial art gymnasiums existing at the time, spun off dissidents that threatened local law and order before government controls could be reinstated. Fortunately, the martial arts of today often act as a filter for those potential ruffians who find the training too extreme and demanding to endure, and the mental requirements far too esoteric. After realizing there are no shortcuts to lasting results, they quickly succumb to failure. By the same token, those seeking skills that can be used primarily in street fighting, but are open to the benefits of spiritual training due to a fundamentally benign nature, become softened and ultimately wiser by the far-reaching effects inherent in traditional taekwondo philosophy.

As a constant reminder of these noble philosophical under-pinnings, the closing ritual in many training halls calls for a recitation of the basic principles that comprise the cornerstone of the Korean martial arts. This present code of honor is directly related to the tenets espoused by the Sesok Ogye bestowed upon the Hwarang-do and remains today as a blueprint for ethical behavior. Not to be construed merely as a neighborly set of val-ues or the casual lines of some benevolent verse, this creed repre-sents a direct link to the past and a reflection of the true essence surrounding the practice of taekwondo.

Taekwondo Code of Honor
(contemporary version)

Be loyal to your country
Be loving and show fidelity to your parents
Be loving between husband and wife
Be cooperative between brothers and sisters
Be faithful to your friends
Be respectful to your elders
Establish trust between teacher and student
Use good judgment before harming any
living thing
Never retreat in battle
Always finish what you start

Having said this, the practitioner may wonder how is it pos-sible to implement such apparently high ideals in a world where we are surrounded by duality and egocentric behavior? Again, drawing on tradition, as did Bodhidharma, we find a possible solution in Buddhist thought. In the practice of Zen, one is constantly reminded to retain *shoshin* or "beginner's mind." We choose to examine this concept here chiefly due to the fact that the "empty" or "innocent" mind of the novice is capable of accepting many more possibilities than that of the expert's which is ostensibly filled with knowledge. Metaphorically speak-ing, the cup that is full needs to be emptied before it can once again be refilled. Therefore, this reference is made in regard to our proclivity for allowing cynicism and complacency to creep into our lives. When applied to the current code of honor, however, the intent of shoshin becomes clear. While simple in nature, the basic precepts of these ethical principles are heavy with meaning and their acceptance, difficult to embrace in the best of times, are mandatory to the proper growth of the martial artist. Subsequently, by reevaluating some of our basic beliefs as seen through the beginner's eye, we may be surprised at the results. For example, we can clearly grasp the value of remaining loyal to our country, but how does this relate to the moral obligation we feel towards our community, home and family? Furthermore, showing love and respect to one's spouse, parents or siblings can easily be taken for granted though with an appreciation of shoshin, methods for improvement may quickly become apparent.

On yet another level, the very nature of the student/teacher relationship dictates that a strong bond of trust be developed so that potentially life threatening techniques may be demonstrated by the instructor on the newcomer without fear of harm. Likewise, the instructor has a moral obligation to the student to guide him properly and patiently on the correct path of the martial arts. The important lesson here is to apply the doctrine of shoshin or "beginner's mind" and innocently, but not blindly, accept these guidelines for what they are—the honorific backbone of traditional taekwondo philosophy. It is essential that the practitioner make every effort to uniquely interpret and apply these values on a daily basis in order to derive the most from his martial arts training. Ingredients of equal importance to the refinement of the taekwondoist are truthfulness, courtesy, loyalty, and restraint. We must be truthful to ourselves and others, show courtesy to those less fortunate than we are, loyalty to the few truly deserving of it, and restraint against using our martial skills for dishonorable causes.

As martial artists and modern day warriors, it is incumbent upon us to act in an honorable manner in setting a worthy example for society at large. It was Confucius who said, "To see what is right and not do it is to want for courage." In taekwondo we actively seek to better our mind and spirit, not simply our physical stature. Subsequently, the cultivation of a noble character typifying honor and respect cannot be ignored. In today's world it is difficult at best to follow our individual sense of honor. Therefore, in embracing the martial arts, we must continue a journey started fourteen hundred years ago, following in the footsteps of the Hwarang warriors and others in their quest for ethical enlightenment.

CHAPTER 4

The Holistic Approach

O ne of the most notable aspects of the martial arts is the attention given to the cultivation of the individual's mind, body, and spirit as a whole. This holistic approach differs greatly from those found in other forms of athletic endeavor and remains the driving force that lies at the heart of traditional taekwondo. Without this unique quality, the martial arts would be considered nothing more than mere sport. To those unfamiliar with this principle, it is assumed that the physical abilities of the participant are of primary concern in developing the skills associated with the martial arts. This notion, however, is inaccurate at best. For those who have devoted their lives to becoming exemplary martial artists, in addition to the obvious physical exercises, have done so through the diligent study of topics such as anatomy, meditation, ethics, healing procedures, pedagogy, nutrition, and Eastern philosophy. By blending these studies with the nurturing of a strong body, a harmonious mixture between fulfillment in life and the martial arts will inevitably result.

Any spectator who has attended a demonstration of the martial arts and seen the dazzling kicks and breaking techniques performed by an experienced martial artist, can bear witness to the fact that physical strength alone would prove inadequate in achieving many of the feats exhibited by the seasoned practitioner. Apart from the entertainment value, the focus and raw will necessary to splinter multiple pieces of wood or stop a kick millimeters from a vital area are born from skills acquired through years of faithful holistic practice. In the early stages of instruction, it is difficult at best for the lower belt to grasp the importance of training in this manner. In their yearning to become virtual copies of their legendary martial arts heroes, the intricacies of taekwondo can be lost. As with any complex form of expression, revelation comes slowly. The image of the martial

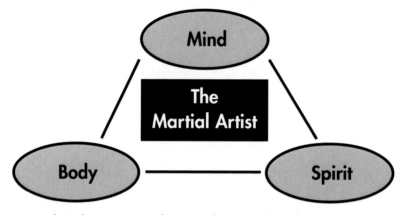

In order to become a complete martial artist mind, body, and spirit must become united as one.

artist portrayed by television, movies, and magazines generates the potential for leaving the newcomer with a false impression of what is actually necessary to gain an acceptable level of proficiency. A great deal of time and energy is required to penetrate the surface of the martial arts in order to discover the benefits this amalgam of mind, body, and spirit has to offer. As with the individual words of a book, one thought leads to another eventually ending in a complete story. The holistic triad of body, mind, and spirit manifests itself in just such a progression. Years may pass before one begins to feel the stirrings of these three basic elements beginning to beat in phase. Patience is required, for it is an appreciation of the process itself that will drive the practitioner forward.

What steps, then, should the newcomer take in his search for a balanced, holistic martial arts training program that will ultimately lead to physical, mental, and spiritual self-fulfillment? To begin with, the first element in the triad, physical fitness, can be attained in a variety of ways. Resistance training, proper nutrition, flexibility training, and aerobic exercise are but a few ways to start on the road to fitness. It is important to note that the dramatic kicks and strikes associated with the art of taekwondo must be executed with explosive force. Since power equals speed plus strength, it is essential that the taekwondoist embark upon a limited program of weight training focusing on leg and arm muscles to achieve this explosiveness. Resistance training in general, as it pertains to the martial arts, has proven to be a source

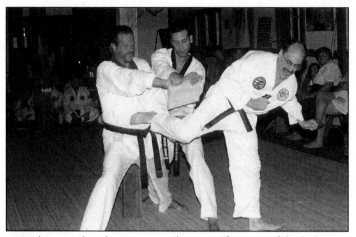

Kyuk Pa or "breaking," is a realistic manifestation of the holistic triad.

of controversy over the years. Claims have been made that bulking up can cause a decrease in speed and flexibility. However, it is commonly recognized today that, in moderation, this form of conditioning is beneficial to cultivate the type of strength necessary to make many of the techniques unique to taekwondo more effective. The type of martial discipline the student has chosen, moreover, will dictate the type of muscle conditioning one should pursue. Judo, for example, would require the development of a different set of muscles then would taijiquan or aikido. The judoka, for instance, must summon up a great deal of upper body strength to complete the throws inherent in that art. Therefore, developing the arm and chest muscles is very important. The aikidoist, on the other hand, must develop an extraordinary sense of balance coupled with the agility to remain unharmed when executing the lock and throw techniques associated with that particular discipline. To the taekwondoist, muscle conditioning plays an essential role because, in its traditional form, taekwondo embraces many of the tactics found in a variety of martial arts. Strength exercises common to most martial arts will include the bench press, butterflies, forearm curls, squats, and leg lifts as well as other related exercises specific to certain muscle groups.

Furthermore, elements common to all martial arts are the need for stamina and flexibility—the ability to twist, kick, throw, and be thrown. The stamina to resist multiple attackers over an extended period of time is also of the utmost importance. These qualities can be realized only through a dedicated program of aerobic exercise. Sprinting, used to develop the fast-twitch muscles, is a particularly worthwhile exercise for the taekwondoist with an eye on competition. Some martial artists have been known to increase lung capacity and heart rate by running up and down stairways of athletic venues. Others turn to rope jumping and heavy bag work as a more traditional source of aerobic exercise. Performing martial arts forms is yet another method of stimulating the respiratory and circulatory systems that will serve the dual purpose of art-specific practice and exercise. Also, we must not lose sight of the fact that the martial arts are extremely demanding on the body's muscular-skeletal structure. It is important that we gain an appreciation for the proper warm up methods used to acclimate these parts of the body. A brief look into the science of sports medicine or the physics of dance can, perhaps, shed some light on these topics. One would think that the time spent in the training hall would be sufficient to meet these demands, but this is simply not true. In the dojang, the practitioner is constantly working on perfecting a variety of new techniques, not necessarily the overt physical characteristics of the body. Subsequently, it is not enough to assume training ends with the removal of the dobok. The *do* in taekwondo signifies that we have begun a journey in pursuit of a way of life. Therefore, the martial artist in search of a holistically disciplined lifestyle should spend time alone expanding the limits of their physical conditioning as well.

Just as we continuously push to expand our physical capabilities, we should also seek methods to expand our mental aptitude. Once we begin stimulating the mind, however, it is important to fill it with topics of a worthwhile nature. As we have seen, the true martial artist should possess a working knowledge of subjects pertinent to his or her chosen discipline. As an example, familiarity with human anatomy becomes essential when one considers that traditional taekwondo doctrine relies heavily on focused strikes to vital areas of the body. A command of the body's pressure points and energy meridians as emphasized in the ancient Chinese art, qigong, can prove invaluable. This is especially true when one considers that the goal of the martial artist is, in most cases, to incapacitate an opponent rather than to seriously injure them. The discipline of qigong also stresses the ability to heal sickness by manipulating ki, the internal life force that resides within all living things. By internally directing the ki to specific areas of need, or externally applying the techniques via accupressure, it is said one can expect relief from illness or injury. This therapeutic system is based on the procedures found in Traditional Chinese Medicine and boasts many documented incidents of success. Possessing these benevolent skills will allow the martial artist to attain equilibrium with nature as dictated by Taoist principle of Yin and Yang—the theory of polar opposites. The martial artist must have the ability to heal, as well as hurt.

If, over the course of our day, we find that we do not have as much time as we would like to devote exclusively to our martial practice, there are other ways we could work in some mental exercise. We might consider reading a book pertaining to our martial art, or playing a game that requires some thought or strategy. Since strategic thinking plays such an important role in the techniques surrounding sport taekwondo, it goes without saying that pursuits of this nature will aid us with our sparring ability. Writing a letter to a friend or, perhaps, learning the language unique to a particular martial art are further methods of "massaging" the brain's gray matter. Just as a body can atrophy with neglect over time, so can an individual's mind. In order to maintain clear thinking and good judgment, one must adhere to a routine of mental exercise. With only twenty-four hours in the day however, when do we find the time to do these things? Consider for a moment the time spent commuting to work or school. Instructional audiocassettes are available that will allow us to use this potentially wasted time more wisely. A by-product of our training is the assumption of a "can do" attitude. It is surprising how one begins to find time for things previously thought impossible to fit in a seemingly full schedule when one truly embraces the way of the martial arts. Presumably, if a daily routine of mental exercise is scheduled and adhered to, before long the student will notice new and worthy habits slowly replacing those of a less desirable nature. Though this growth may not be fully self-evident. It will more likely reveal itself to an acquaintance or relative the practitioner has not seen for some time. This distant friend will most certainly notice a beneficial change or difference in the practitioner's overall demeanor.

When following the holistic approach inherent in taekwondo, priority must be assigned to nurturing the spiritual aspect of the art in concert with the mental and physical elements. One tool that can be used in tilling the soil of the soul is meditation. Unfortunately, meditation is an often-overlooked practice in modern taekwondo, but it remains a vital part of the martial artist's holistic development. Eastern thought stresses the importance of mind and body unification in the martial arts. One method of achieving this seemingly elusive characteristic is through the intense mental focus inspired by the practice of meditation. Since the body is controlled by the mind, it follows that all the strength gained through physical conditioning is worthless without the will to implement it. Searching through history we find numerous tales of the meek dominating the strong by trusting in the confidence forged by an iron will. Subsequently, by practicing meditation along with cultivating virtues such as indomitable spirit, confidence, and courage—virtues that set the martial artist apart from the street brawler—the practitioner's technique will be that much more effective. Furthermore, the relaxation, release, and reflective qualities offered by the sincere practice of meditation could have a major effect on the way we view our lives and ourselves in general.

Taekwondo is known for its dramatic techniques and one method in particular that has traditionally tested all three elements of the holistic triad is *kyuk pa* or breaking. Korean taekwondo is not the only martial art to use this technique to gauge the practitioner's holistic prowess. It is through the practice of *tameshiwari* (to test while breaking), that proponents of Japanese *karate* and practitioners of the *Koei-Kan* system, in particular, establish a measure of confidence and spiritual fortitude. The evolution of this practice can be traced back centuries to the study of *kenjutsu* (swordsmanship) where the Japanese samurai would test their technique and the sharpness of their blades by striking cadavers. Today, breaking techniques pervade many of the martial arts in an effort to test the student's concentration and focus. The ability to break, while made to look simple, requires a great deal of courage and respect for the object to be broken. The martial artist must approach the board or brick with only one thought in mind—that the hand will pass through the object as if there were no opportunity for failure— that, essentially, the deed has already been done. It is with this mental image derived from a display of indomitable spirit and extreme focus that success is assured. Imagine approaching every obstacle in life with equal vigor!

It is unfortunate, to say the least, when those initially exploring the martial arts turn away without ever realizing or being told of a discipline's true intent. A perfunctory glance will never reveal the great gift of fulfillment bestowed by merging the mind, body, and soul through diligent, holistic training. As we have come to see however, the ultimate goal of taekwondo is the individual's total self-improvement with equal attention given to the practitioner's physical, mental, and spiritual health. Consequently, it is gratifying indeed when the student senses a ripple in the muscle of confidence or a tightening in the sinews of self-esteem. This, coupled with the emotional stability one will surely come to enjoy in the long term, is reward enough for the long hours invested in this wholesome exercise. The spiritual, mental, and physical value gained from a true holistic approach to living can have profound effects not only on ourselves, but also on those around us. Sadly, in their desperate search for internal peace, a growing component of today's global society has turned to drugs or alcohol as an artificial means of pacification. Temporary in nature, these substances can never replace the true remedies necessary to achieve genuine self-enlightenment. Although it is unrealistic to assume direct responsibility for the betterment of the world population as a whole, it is possible to begin, on a manageable level, by focusing on one's own world view. Peace radiates outward—first from the individual, then to the family, followed by the community and ultimately, society at large. While the martial arts do not profess to be a panacea for the ills of mankind, they can offer hope for those prepared to bring the holistic triad into balance.

Chapter 5
The Enemy Within

Proficiency in the martial arts does not come easy. If it did, everyone would rush to become a martial artist. The desire to defend ourselves in sensitive situations, whether it is verbally with confidence or physically with technique, is something we all have in common. As with any worthwhile endeavor however, it requires work—hard work not only of a physical nature, but on a mental and emotional level as well. The last thing many of us wish to do after a particularly trying day at home or in the office, is begin a routine of physical exercise. We feel we have put in our time for the day and now it is time to relax. This is understandable, but those of us who aspire to become competent martial artists realize that this added effort is exactly what is required. Not surprisingly, given the chemical reactions that take place in the body following a strenuous workout, we actually feel better for it. However, the thought of what comes after does not necessarily make up for what comes before. It is situations such as these that distinguish the true martial artist from the daydreamer.

When we look in the mirror, the image we perceive is a reflection of the person we've created in our mind. Our persona is (in addition to a multitude of other psychological and physical factors) a product of the manner in which we were raised, our physical appearance, the criticism we receive from others, and our successes and failures. Furthermore, it is difficult, if not impossible, for us to remain genuinely objective regarding our self-image. To dwell too long on this topic can result in either conceit or despair. Suffice it to say that, given the wide spectrum of emotional possibilities we are capable of, we should not be overly critical of ourselves. Rather, we should concentrate on developing our strengths while transforming, fortifying, and eliminating our weaknesses.

Countless times during our lives we have heard the phrase,

"We are our own worst enemy." For many of us, this thought rings true. How many times have we put off a chore we would rather not do, or have given up on a task that appears too difficult to complete? As we have seen, the art of taekwondo, by virtue of its ethical code of behavior, aggressively encourages tenacity and perseverance. The tenets, never retreat in battle and always finish what you start, are signposts that, when construed in the proper frame of mind, point the way to avoiding laziness and procrastination. For example, in the early stages of training, the physical aspect of taekwondo assumes center stage and begins to dominate the practitioner's way of thinking. This is a dangerous time in that many cannot see beyond it, and quickly become discouraged. Sore muscles and limited endurance become worthy opponents in our battle against failure. This is especially true for the participant that becomes involved at an advanced stage of life. The self-doubt we experience when faced with the athletically gifted student who performs a perfect split or jumping technique is a common response shared by all at one time or another. We must remind ourselves, in instances such as these, that ultimately we are competing against ourselves rather than others. This is clearly one of the first lessons the novice martial artist must embrace in order to continue training in a positive fashion.

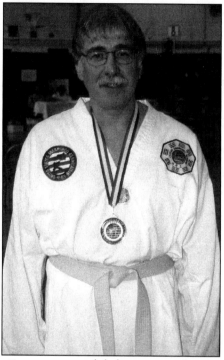

Perseverance and dedication are allies in the battle against the "enemy within." The rewards are great for the taekwondo student who practices these virtues.

Once this is fully understood, our resolve can be trusted to carry us forward. Martial arts techniques, while made to look simple when executed by an accomplished practitioner, are everything but simple! A veteran modern dance instructor once commented that, "Teaching the mind a step or movement is easy. It is inculcating the muscle fibers and joints with this memory that is the difficult part." This two-step approach to learning any physical technique involving muscle memory is a lesson students at all levels would do well to bear in mind.

Forms or poom-se training is a good place to put the above belief of personal competition into practice. Forms are combinations of choreographed techniques aimed at defeating multiple opponents attacking from various directions. Students often have a habit of stealing a glance at one another during class in hopes of confirming that their own movements within a given poom-se are correct. Realizing that this segment of our training is an iteration of moving meditation, it is essential that students remain focused on their own movements. In most cases the techniques are usually executed in an acceptable fashion until the student's confidence falters and their concentration is broken. Assuming the practitioner has allowed the motions of a given form to become ingrained through constant practice, he should not permit himself to become distracted by external diversions (in this case, the surrounding environment or fellow students) and trust in his own abilities. In an effort to confront this "breach of concentration," some schools have instituted the practice of performing forms in directions other than those with which students are most familiar. Simple in nature, this method of instruction serves the dual purpose of forcing the issues of attentiveness and focus, so sorely needed in dealing with foreign situations while nurturing the principle of personal competition. What, one may ask, does this have to do with applying martial arts philosophy to daily life? Clearly, the freedoms we enjoy as citizens of a great nation is something we all hold dear. However, our ability to focus can sometimes be confounded given the enormity of choice we are privileged with. Which way do we turn when given an option? What car should we drive? Which clothes should we wear? The hope is that eventually these lessons, attributed to taekwondo training, will be utilized and carried over into the student's daily routine allowing them to more sharply focus on the choices they are faced with.

Yet another arena in the martial arts where we fall victim to the enemy within, is that of contact sparring. Unlike modern forms of pugilism, the martial arts in general and sport taekwondo in particular, demand more than a modicum of respect between competitors. Thrown into a ring, any able bodied person can seriously injure another by indiscriminately kicking and punching without restraint or focus. This is clearly not the intent of the martial artist. However, staring into the eyes of an unknown competitor clad in regulation fighting gear can fill the heart of many with fear and apprehension. Unbeknownst to the novice, this is a symptom shared by everyone from the most experienced tournament fighter to the lower belt donning a *hogu* (chest protector) for the first time. It is fairly safe to assume that most human beings inherently do not enjoy having blows rain down upon them. The fear we feel is a manifestation of our basic, primordial instinct for self-preservation. It is the brain's method of signaling us to remain alert for potential danger and any attempt to short circuit this emotion by ignoring it could have disastrous consequences.

Fear triggers our body's defense mechanism by introducing physiological changes that result in, among other things, an acute awareness of our surroundings. This heightened state of consciousness is a condition referred to by some as being "battle bright." In this state, vision sharpens, the auditory and olfactory senses are amplified, and our reaction time increases. Once in

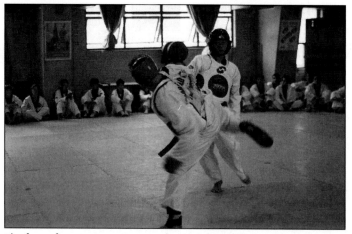

The fear of contact sparring can be transformed into a positive experience through strategic thinking.

this condition, we are more apt to become aware of our opponent's body language. In many instances an individual will telegraph an incoming technique by a certain facial expression or stance. At this point, the student should react quickly, snatching the opportunity to defend with a counterattack quickly followed by an offensive strike drawn from his own arsenal of techniques. This strategy typifies the traditional taekwondo principle of defend and attack as dictated by the Yin/Yang. (Um/Yang in Korean.) Additionally, part of the success in overcoming the fear of sparring is hidden in the fact that the student has been trained in the physical vocabulary of the art and any responsible instructor would not permit entrance into the ring without this knowledge. Viewed in this light, fear can become an ally rather than a foe in our quest for victory over ourselves as well as our opponents. In reality, it is far more likely that the "matches" we encounter everyday will be on an emotional, intellectual, or verbal basis rather than on a physical plane. When a situation arises where our anxiety begins to take control, we must recall the lessons we have learned and use them to our advantage in our daily lives, as well as in the ring.

On the other hand, as we have seen earlier, many individuals turn to the martial arts in search of discipline. The martial arts have a great deal to do with discipline, and its proper application can have far reaching consequences on controlling the enemy within. Without discipline, it is nearly impossible to exorcise internal turmoil and increase our sense of self-esteem. In today's society, we are witnessing an alarming deterioration of moral values. What was once considered unthinkable is now nearly commonplace. Whether this decline can be attributed to the continuing breakup of the family unit, or the average citizen's avoidance of ethical mores, is not to be debated here. A conclusion can be drawn however that the lack of discipline we are presently experiencing runs parallel to these trends.

Taekwondo has become an answer to the woes of many parents seeking to instill discipline and a robust set of moral values in their children without the dogma typically associated with religion. Likewise, adults find the highly structured routines intrinsic to taekwondo appealing to their fundamental need for ritualized activities. One cannot survive in the martial arts without a strict adherence to discipline. Upon enrolling, the new student is immediately familiarized with the proper etiquette that will be expected of them. Caring for their dobok, bowing correctly, the show of respect for seniors, are essential to the martial tradition. By allowing humility to become the medium in which discipline can germinate and prosper, the martial artist will harvest a newly found sense of self-esteem that will act as a fortification against the enemy within. The manifestations of these attributes will not only show themselves in the student's technique, but in the way they carry themselves as well. Moreover, as the individual progresses through the ranks, he comes to realize that the discipline gleaned from taekwondo training is so imbued in his life, that almost without his knowledge, he begins to exhibit its benefits in everyday life.

It is unlikely that Bodhidharma and the members of the Hwarang could have foreseen the remedial effects their art would have in our effort to silence our internal demons. But suffice it to say that even they must have suffered from self-doubt at one time or another. It must be remembered that, for hundreds of years, although there existed the underlying intention of addressing social issues, the martial arts were primarily taught as a weapon of war. Fortunately for us today, in addition to being a means of self-defense, the maturation process that has occurred over the centuries has brought with it a blueprint which we can pattern our lives after and in doing so, gain victory over the enemy within.

CHAPTER 6

Measurable Goals

It is not uncommon for the beginner martial artist to feel frustrated when faced with what appears to be a never-ending arsenal of stances, kicks, strikes, and blocks. As if the sheer quantity of these techniques alone were not enough to create anguish, with each new class the novice runs the risk of being exposed to students who, by virtue of age, gender, or tenure, often possess superior form, stamina, or skill. If the aspirant were to view this vast landscape of knowledge without considering the milestones along the way, the task of learning could potentially become overwhelming. As with any journey however, it is difficult to arrive at a point of destination without realizing ahead of time where you are going. Likewise, any arduous adventure must begin with the first step and include places to stop and rest for reflection along the way. Imagine attempting a drive across the country without stopping for gasoline or sleep! Clearly, one would not get very far.

As we have come to see, taekwondo is not a static achievement, but a dynamic journey fraught with experiences as diverse as any one would come to expect from a prolonged artistic expression of this nature. Morihei Ueshiba, the father of Japanese aikido, was known to have said in his later years, "This old man is still learning." Therefore, it would indeed be counterproductive for the novice to make the mistaken assumption that earning a black belt signals the completion of their training. Consequently, once one comes to grips with the concept that any serious study of the martial arts is a lifelong pursuit, they must then set short-, as well as long-term goals, in order to achieve observable results. It is of the utmost importance that these goals are both attainable and measurable in order to avoid succumbing to a sense of futility.

We are allotted only a certain amount of time on this earth to achieve the goals we set for ourselves. Furthermore, if we spend this time foolishly fretting over the amount of time or effort it may take to complete a project, we may never accomplish anything at all. Attempting too much too soon clearly presents the potential for discouragement and ultimately, failure. Instead we should partition our tasks, whether they are at work, school, or the dojang, into manageable parcels. This is especially true in situations that call for extreme patience and concentration. As with the reformed alcoholic who tests his sobriety on a day-to-day basis, certain situations in life call for this time-apportioned approach—an approach that offers foreseeable, rewarding results in the short term. It is often easier to understand and retain information if it is taken in small, digestible portions rather than in one large dose. This is the course one should chart in any worthy study of the martial arts. In taekwondo, these essential goals are characterized and quantified by a system of belt promotions. Learning to cope with a particularly stressful, long term situation in life, or simply striving for something that may require a great deal of effort over an extended period of time can have much in common with earning the various belts associated with the martial arts.

While there are inherent differences according to the art in question, most martial disciplines today traditionally adhere to some type of formal ranking system. Typically, these grades are signified by different color belts so as to distinguish between the novice and the student who has gained a higher degree of proficiency. While the belt itself is meaningless without the knowledge to back it up, it is sometimes regarded as a reward unto itself. The belt system is a tangible indication to the world of the student's determination and will to move forward, sometimes in the face of extreme physical adversity. It should be noted that in the early phase of martial arts development, there existed only two belts— white and black. The creation of this multi-colored, belt ranking system is attributed to both General Choi, founder of the International Taekwondo Federation and contributor to the name taekwondo itself, and Jigoro Kano, the father of Japanese judo. Furthermore, the representative color of these belts is not arbitrary. They each have a set philosophy congruent with the growth of the individual.

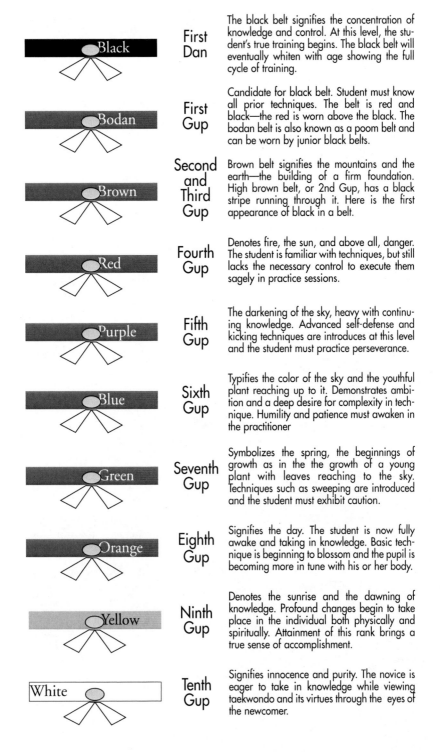

First Dan — The black belt signifies the concentration of knowledge and control. At this level, the student's true training begins. The black belt will eventually whiten with age showing the full cycle of training.

First Gup — Candidate for black belt. Student must know all prior techniques. The belt is red and black—the red is worn above the black. The bodan belt is also known as a poom belt and can be worn by junior black belts.

Second and Third Gup — Brown belt signifies the mountains and the earth—the building of a firm foundation. High brown belt, or 2nd Gup, has a black stripe running through it. Here is the first appearance of black in a belt.

Fourth Gup — Denotes fire, the sun, and above all, danger. The student is familiar with techniques, but still lacks the necessary control to execute them sagely in practice sessions.

Fifth Gup — The darkening of the sky, heavy with continuing knowledge. Advanced self-defense and kicking techniques are introduces at this level and the student must practice perseverance.

Sixth Gup — Typifies the color of the sky and the youthful plant reaching up to it. Demonstrates ambition and a deep desire for complexity in technique. Humility and patience must awaken in the practitioner

Seventh Gup — Symbolizes the spring, the beginnings of growth as in the the growth of a young plant with leaves reaching to the sky. Techniques such as sweeping are introduced and the student must exhibit caution.

Eighth Gup — Signifies the day. The student is now fully awake and taking in knowledge. Basic technique is beginning to blossom and the pupil is becoming more in tune with his or her body.

Ninth Gup — Denotes the sunrise and the dawning of knowledge. Profound changes begin to take place in the individual both physically and spiritually. Attainment of this rank brings a true sense of accomplishment.

Tenth Gup — Signifies innocence and purity. The novice is eager to take in knowledge while viewing taekwondo and its virtues through the eyes of the newcomer.

In modern martial arts culture, a great deal of reverence and importance is associated with the earning of a black belt. In the eyes of many, the holder takes on a mystical quality propagated by Asian martial lore. Any candidate whose primary goal is simply to wear the black belt however, is in for a rude awakening. Statistically, two out of every one hundred individuals who begin martial arts training graduate to black belt! Why is this ratio so slim? The reality of the situation becomes evident when one considers the effort and perseverance it takes to achieve this, the ultimate of measurable goals in the martial arts. Ideally, belts of any color are not given out freely, but are granted according to the practitioner's capabilities. Elevation in status is predicated on the student mastering a given set of required techniques at each subsequent level. In addition to being conversant in martial philosophy and exuding the proper attitude, the taekwondo student must demonstrate advanced technical abilities in a poom-se or hyung form, self-defense (*ho shin sul*), one-step sparring (*il su shik*), free sparring (*kyorugi*) and breaking (*kyuk pa*) in order to qualify for the next belt. As the student progresses, they test their abilities before a panel of judges who will ultimately determine if a promotion in rank is warranted. Generally, the student is allowed to advance at his or her own pace. However, the majority of dojangs offer promotion examinations every few months. At this rate, a student of taekwondo can theoretically attain black belt status within three years.

A typical martial arts curriculum is constructed in such a way so as to encourage the student by increasing self-esteem as they gain proficiency. This would not be possible if the student left the dojang every time feeling he had accomplished nothing. This goal is achieved by bringing the practitioner up to the black belt level by degrees rather than in one large leap. This is the concept behind dividing our efforts into discrete blocks of knowledge. We are then afforded the luxury of focusing on only those techniques applicable to the given belt level. This is not to say that our previous lessons should be stored away and forgotten. On the contrary, each piece of the puzzle should be held firmly in place until the total picture finally comes into view.

Moreover, every day we see new students eager to begin training in taekwondo. At the start it is something new and exciting in their life. Many confess that they have secretly desired to become involved in the martial arts for many years. However, by the end of their first class they almost always appear somewhat flustered and confused. Not only can they not recall the basic warm-up exercises, but they can hardly remember the fundamental stances they have just been shown. This is normal and must be expected. There are many routines and rituals one needs to become accustomed to in the dojang environment. For example, most Westerners tend to exhibit some difficulty with the concept of bowing to their instructors and other seniors in the early phases of their training. In addition, while many students have no problem speaking loudly outside the training hall, once inside, timidity steps in and they suddenly loose the ability to emit the *kihop* or spirit yell so essential to the proper execution of taekwondo techniques. However, once the novice acclimates to and moves beyond these fundamental procedures, their education takes on a more routine complexion. This is the stage at which goal setting becomes paramount. The dynamics of achieving a goal or rank has the motivating effect of making the student want to go further. When one obstacle is overcome, the student becomes aware of the fact that he has advanced that much further along and is prepared to tackle the next hurdle towards total self-improvement. This is a major consideration in attaining success on the road to a black belt.

In my own experience, upon completion of a particularly grueling belt test, I was once criticized by one of the presiding masters of the event as having an ill-defined front kick (*ap chagi*.) After some initial frustration, I quickly recovered after realizing that there was some validity in his remark. At that moment, rather than becoming discouraged, I set a goal for myself to develop what I hoped would be an exemplary, head level front kick worthy of future comment. Each day thereafter, upon entering the dojang, I would assume a fighting stance (kyoreugi jase), while watching in the mirror to monitor my progress. To a four-count, I would first lift my right leg, chambering my knee, then extend my lower leg, holding it out while pointing with the ball of my foot (*ap chook*) at an imaginary target. Next, I would lower my leg with my knee remaining in the chambered position. At the count of four I would return to the fighting stance and begin again. After repeating this exercise in slow motion almost daily for a period of two months, I began to notice an improvement. With each successive attempt, I began to raise the kick up by inches, until today, I feel I have achieved an element of success. Had I started out attempting to kick as high as possible, the task may have been that much more difficult. By breaking it down, executing the kicks in slow motion, my leg grew stronger still and the technique improved over time.

In today's complex world it is very easy to become overwhelmed by a variety of circumstances. Financial obligations, business negotiations, even schoolwork for the young, can take on enormous proportions when viewed in their entirety. Of course, a key element in the successful implementation of this chapter's concept is patience. Without it one cannot expect to persevere and realize results. However, by applying the principle of measurable goals gleaned from martial arts training, we may be better prepared to cope with what may initially appear to be insurmountable obstacles.

CHAPTER 7

Poom-Se: Moving Meditation

The martial arts are rich in traditions that date back thousands of years with roots deep in Asian philosophy. One such tradition that defines the physical, spiritual and aesthetic dimensions of taekwondo in particular, is the practice of poom-se or forms. Poom-se are choreographed combinations of techniques, aimed at defeating imaginary opponents attacking from multiple directions. To the eye of the uninitiated, these motions may appear somewhat like the movements of a dance. In his book, *The Making of a Martial Artist*, Grand Master Sang Kyu Shim supports this notion by comparing the martial artist more to a ballet dancer than a boxer. But make no mistake, for while this analogy suggests the poise, grace, and agility common to the two, that is where the similarity ends. Form practice represents the essence of the fighting arts, allowing the student to execute the techniques they have learned in an organized, forceful manner.

Form training lends a unique identity to a given martial art whether it is taekwondo, taijiquan, or karate and constitutes a large segment of its curriculum. Hence, in his definitive volume, *Tae Kwon Do: A Korean Martial Art*, Grand Master Richard Chun states categorically that, "Without forms there is no taekwondo." Consequently, it is widely accepted that adherence to these forms differentiate traditional martial art from martial sport. An observation by a noted instructor confirms this theory when he states that anyone can learn to kick and punch, but it is the poom-se that earns the belt. Mastering a given poom-se demands the student repeat the successive motions hundreds of times. It is through diligent practice and repetition that the inherent techniques become branded upon the student's subconscious memory resulting in an instinctive response should a situation requiring defensive measures arise. This is the first step in executing the form with power, grace, and fluidity.

The elements that compose a poom-se are not arbitrary. They are believed to have been devised in ancient times as a method for victorious warriors returning from combat to demonstrate tried and true techniques to younger recruits eager for battle. A seasoned soldier of the Hwarang, for example, may have demonstrated to a comrade how he deflected an incoming blow by utilizing what we have come to know as a middle block (*momtang makki*) quickly followed by a reverse or high punch, punctuated by a loud kihop. He would then spin around executing a comparable strategy at yet another attacker. Conceivably, once the survivability value in this type of training became apparent, it was embellished upon to include more advanced and complex combinations of techniques. Confirmation of this belief can be seen in

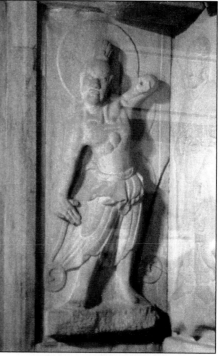

A stone likeness of the ancient warrior, Kumgang Yuksa, guarding the Buddha at Sokkuram Grotto, Korea.

the form of the great warrior Kumgang Yuksa whose likeness stands chiseled in the stone walls of Sokkuram Grotto in Kyongju. There he has stood for centuries protecting the entrance, poised in a fighting stance displaying a high, rising block in conjunction with a low, side block (*yop makki*). Furthermore, history supports the theory that it was through execution of poom-se that great masters of the past, living a life of solitude in Buddhist temples, would practice the dynamic movements of their art in order to cultivate a strong body and disciplined mind. In the case of Bodhidharma and his disciples

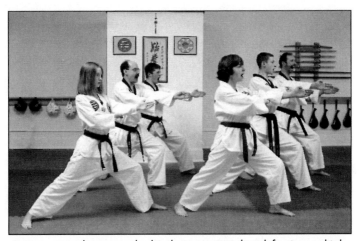

Poom-se are choreographed techniques aimed at defeating multiple attackers coming from various directions.

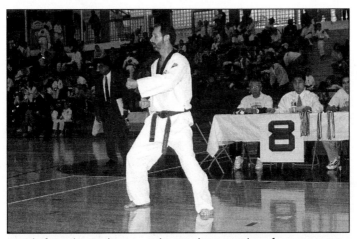

Aside from the meditative and strengthening value of poom-se, it is also practiced in tournament competition.

at the Shaolin temple, form practice was used not only as a blueprint for transmission of their art, but also as a method of exercise and internal energy (ki) development. It is through the execution of poom-se, therefore, that the dynamic movements of what we know today as taekwondo have been handed down from generation to generation.

It must be remembered that until the latter part of the twentieth century, full contact sparring did not exist either as a sport or training procedure. This was partially due to the lack

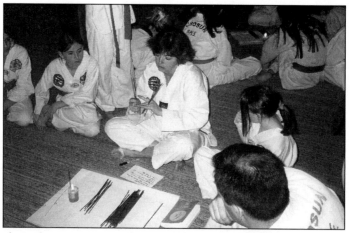

of
The I Ching is an Asian classic and has been used for centuries as a method of forecasting future events. Here, students manipulate yarrow stalks in an effort to understand the underlying philosophy of the I Ching.

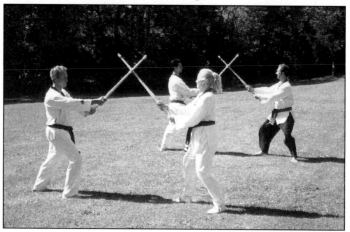

Taekwondo students practicing a sword poom-se.

adequate protective equipment coupled with the fact that the martial arts were primarily intended as a means of self-defense. Techniques were taught to be practiced full force, stopping inches short of their intended target. Today, with taekwondo rapidly becoming a prominent martial sport, many students are sadly turning their backs on traditional form training, unable to grasp the worth of what is essentially the soul of the martial arts. This symptom is painfully apparent among those who, as a

famous meditation teacher once wrote, are "willing to do anything for their advancement except work for it." When one considers the manifold benefits hidden beneath the surface, however,
the value of poom-se training becomes abundantly clear. The
practice of poom-se, among other things, increases the student's
ability to focus and concentrate. It must be remembered that the
primary concern in form training is to defend against multiple
attackers. It is essential, therefore, that we practice aiming our
techniques at precise target areas while simultaneously applying
the proper amount of force necessary to incapacitate an imaginary opponent. The body must remain relaxed until the moment
of impact when all our internal energy is focused on a single
point in space in order to achieve maximum effect thus reflecting
Um/Yang philosophy. This ability to focus so thoroughly can
prove highly beneficial when we find ourselves in a situation that
demands our total concentration in daily life.

Furthermore, while we always seem to favor one side of our
body over the other, the practice of poom-se, by virtue of the lines
of motion, often results in muscular development and dexterity in
both the right and left sides of the body. Many of the techniques
are actually mirror images of one another since we are constantly
changing direction in order to confront yet another imaginary
assailant. This can benefit those with certain physical disabilities
that might otherwise require tedious and often painful physical
therapy. By the same token, on a purely physical level, by infusing
the proper rhythm and strength necessary to make the
movements effective, the practitioner is also performing an
intense aerobic exercise. After many repetitions day after day, a
pronounced increase in stamina cannot help but manifest itself.
The practitioner, due to physical as well as spiritual considerations, should never attempt to perform a poom-se other than one
with which they have been gifted without the express permission
of their instructor. Moreover, each poom-se should be regarded as
a single, living entity unique to the student's current abilities and
not viewed merely as a combination of kicks and punches. With
this in mind, an individual poom-se can be thought of as a single
volume in a set of encyclopedia to be brought down from the
shelf when a certain technique or movement needs to be refer-
enced. Poom-se should not be performed in a robotic fashion but

executed in a pattern of sequences rather than to a standard count. Likewise, it is equally important to exercise proper breath control during poom-se practice. By synchronizing one's inhalations and exhalations to the various motions, the practitioner will appear relaxed and at ease, adding to the aesthetic quality of the form. It is said that many Westerners do not breathe correctly, and have a tendency to gulp shallow quantities of air rather than using a deep, prolonged rhythmic approach to respiration. Correct breathing during poom-se practice has the added benefit of filling the body's core with much needed oxygen and ridding it of carbon dioxide and other toxins. By breathing deeply, using the diaphragm, we are also massaging our internal organs. Many Asian and East Indian beliefs regarding deep breathing center on the fact that the air we breathe contains a life-giving spiritual ingredient known as *prana*. Consequently, the deeper we breathe, the more prana we are taking in. This concept is consistent with a belief in ki, as seen in other Asian cultures.

Performed by an accomplished martial artist, a poom-se is a magnificent sight to behold. Once, while training in Korea, I had the pleasure of experiencing a demonstration of this nature. We were traveling north on the Korean peninsula when we pulled into a rest stop along the highway. Being a red belt at the time, my rank required that I learn the form, *Taegeuk Chil Jang.* Standing in the parking lot, adjacent to our tour bus, Grand Master Yoon Jai Cho, a renowned Korean martial artist graced us with a stunning performance of this poom-se. At one point, the surrounding area echoed with the slap of flesh upon flesh as the sole of his foot came up to meet the palm of his hand in what appeared to be a perfect crescent kick (*pyojak chagi*). With strength and agility, he continued moving from stance to stance displaying both beauty and grace until, upon completion, he returned to the ready (joon-bi) stance.

Needless to say, there have been many iterations of poom-se developed over the years with each master interpreting a form differently, adding his or her own distinctive flavor to the motions. Some dojangs may incorporate forms originating from other disciplines or create their own altogether. Others, with a measure of controversy, put forms to music. Even Korea itself is not immune to this trend where poom-se, aerobics, and dance are blended together to create the new gymnastic art form, *tae kwon che jo*. Moreover, in researching the lineage of taekwondo poom-se, we find a direct link to those practiced during the 1940's and 50's when the art bore the name of *kong soo do* (empty hand way). Subsequently, many of the more advanced poom-se still being taught today are, in some cases, direct decedents of Shotokan/Shorei-ryu karatedo forms (*kata*). This is not at all surprising when one considers the extent of Japanese influence on the martial arts during the long years of occupation between 1910 and 1945. Poom-se such as *Bassai, Jion, Jitte,* and the *Kicho* series continue to be deeply embedded in the traditional way of teaching regardless of pedigree. In answer to the growing popularity of taekwondo, the World Taekwondo Federation, headquartered at the Kukkiwon in Seoul with a membership of nearly fifty million, has chosen to exclusively recognize only certain sets of poom-se, tying each to a successive belt rank. Consequently, in an effort to maintain uniformity, the WTF has officially sanctioned approximately twenty-four poom-se for use in affiliated dojangs and at tournaments throughout the world. Furthermore, it should be noted that the assignment of these various forms among the ascending belt levels might differ somewhat from school to school. Most dojangs, however, have conformed to a standard system of poom-se consistent with rank advancement.

In some cases, the eight *Palgwe* forms supplant or reinforce the Taegeuk series as the required poom-se for color belt promotion. The Palgwe forms, being of a more traditional nature, feature lower stances, and emphasize a greater amount of hand techniques. The Taegeuk series, conversely, were developed later and stress upright-fighting stances more in line with modern sparring strategy. It should be noted that the decision to avoid using WTF forms within a curriculum in no way reflects adversely on a school's traditional validity. This is particularly evident in the forms practiced by the International Taekwondo Federation under the direction of General Choi Hong Hi, which, in contrast, are radically different from those sanctioned by the WTF. As stated earlier, however, some masters have chosen to integrate or continue using traditional poom-se created prior to the birth of the WTF in 1973. Some of these bear the signature of *Moo Duk*

TAEKWONDO POOM-SE

SERIES	POOM-SE		PHILOSOPHY	
KICHO 1-3	Kicho Il Kicho Ee Kicho Sam		Foundation, Beginning or Circle of Life	
TAEGUEK 1-8	Taeguek Il Jang Taeguek Ee Jang Taeguek Sam Jang Taeguek Sa Jang Taeguek Oh Jang Taeguek Yook Jang Taeguek Chil Jang Taeguek Pal Jang		Heaven and Light Joy or Lake Fire and Sun Thunder Wind Water Mountain Earth	
PALGWE 1-8	Palgwe Il Jang Palgwe Ee Jang Palgwe Sam Jang Palgwe Sa Jang Palgwe Oh Jang Palgwe Yook Jang Palgwe Chil Jang Palgwe Pal Jang		Law or Command of the Universe	
WTF BLACK BELT	Koryo Keumgang Taebaek Pyongwon Sipjin Jitae Cheonkwon Hansoo Ilyo		Korea Diamond Mountain Plain Decimal Earth Sky Water Oneness	
MDK Moo Duk Kwan **ITF** International TKD Federation	Tigil 1-2 Chul Ki 1-3 Yunbee Chintae Jion Bal Sek	Kibon 1-5 Chon Ji Dan Gun Do San Won Hyo Yul Gok	Joong Gun Toi Gye Hwarang	

Kwan/Tang Soo Do poom-se for instance. Others may actually be of Japanese or Chinese origin. Ultimately, however, it is of the utmost importance to recall that the performance of poom-se is a vital link to the past and must be practiced diligently if one truly wishes to become proficient in a given martial art.

In addition to improving focus, concentration, speed, and stamina, taekwondo poom-se reflect specific philosophies that can easily be applied to situations that arise in daily life. It is important, however, that we first appreciate the source from which these philosophies derive. Some five thousand years ago, it is said that the Taoist sage, Fu Hsi (2953-2838 BCE), composed what is commonly accepted today as the most ancient of Chinese writings, the *I Ching* or *The Book of Changes*. This classic, amended by Confucius, was considered an oracle a source of advice for those seeking direction in business, politics, and life in general. The formula for use of this compendium is based largely upon the duality of opposites or the Yin/Yang (Um/Yang in Korean). The Yin/Yang is further sub-divided into eight trigrams, subsequently followed by sixty-four hexagrams, thus giving us the final tools necessary to manipulate the I Ching. If one were to examine the original eight trigrams however, he would discover a direct correlation between their meanings, and those philosophies that lie behind the eight Tageuk and Palgwe poom-se.

POOM-SE PHILOSOPHY

Poom-se: Taegeuk Il Jang
Trigram: ☰
I Ching Interpretation: Sky
Taegeuk Interpretation: Heaven and Light
Taegeuk Philosophy: This is the concept of pure Yang. It is the creative force associated with Heaven and Light— the beginning, the creation.

Poom-se: Taegeuk Yee Jang
Trigram: ☱
I Ching Interpretation: Lake
Taegeuk Interpretation: Joy
Taegeuk Philosophy: This is joy. It represents something of a

spiritually uplifting nature. Not aggressive, it is serene and gentle, like bubbles flowing to the surface of a lake.

Poom-se: Taegeuk Sam Jang

Trigram: ☲

I Ching Interpretation: Fire

Taegeuk Interpretation: Fire and Sun

Taegeuk Philosophy: This means Fire and Sun, so the movements of this form must emulate the qualities of fire— a flickering energy of unpredictable pace and styling, and of quiet followed by great excitement or great passion. Something that is continually moving and burning.

Poom-se: Taegeuk Sa Jang

Trigram: ☳

I Ching Interpretation: Thunder

Taegeuk Interpretation: Thunder

Taegeuk Philosophy: Symbolizes Thunder, suggesting courage in the face of danger, as the element of fear and trembling occasionally enters our lives. This form expresses fear in the only way that virtue can—as a passing thunderstorm that nourishes the soul. Virtue, therefore, defines fear as courage.

Poom-se: Taegeuk Oh Jang

Trigram: ☴

I Ching Interpretation: Wind

Taegeuk Interpretation: Wind

Taegeuk Philosophy: Symbolizes Wind. It is sometimes gentle, sometimes forceful, yielding and penetrating, soothing and destructive, invisible, yet manifesting. Interplay of Um and Yang taking place.

Poom-se: Taegeuk Yook Jang

Trigram: ☵

I Ching Interpretation: Water

Taegeuk Interpretation: Water

Taegeuk Philosophy: This means Water and represents the characteristics of consistency and flow. It is to be recognized as a type of confidence where one is able to meet difficulties in life and overcome them, as long as one retains the qualities of acceptance, flow, and natural integrity.

Poom-se: Taegeuk Chil Jang
Trigram: ☶
I Ching Interpretation: Mountain
Taegeuk Interpretation: Top Stop
Taegeuk Philosophy: This suggests the wisdom of knowing when and where to stop—as if one were traveling up a steep mountain. This form interprets the dual principles of stability and ambition.

Poom-se: Taegeuk Pal Jang
Trigram: ☷
I Ching Interpretation: Earth
Taegeuk Interpretation: Earth
Taegeuk Philosophy: Concept of pure Um. The opposite of Taegeuk's first form, it symbolizes the yielding Earth that provides the substance and limitations into which the forces of creation pass to produce physical form. It represents the Mother, checking on all prior learning.

The student of taekwondo may be surprised at the value contained in the application of traditional poom-se philosophy as it applies to particular sets of circumstances that may arise in daily life. For instance, *Taegeuk Yook Jang,* meaning Water, focuses on our ability to overcome life's hardships through the virtue of acceptance and flow. Water in a stream does not force its way through a rock, but rather travels around it, eventually wearing it down in the process. This lesson can prove highly beneficial in coping with difficulties requiring patience and tenacity in daily life. In fact, *hapkido,* a related Korean martial art, as well as aikido, the Japanese discipline, are founded on this very principle of acceptance and flow. By blending with, rather than resisting an attack, the aggressor's negative energy is reflected and used as a weapon against him, thus betraying him in the process. Similarly, *Taegeuk Oh Jang,* represented by Wind, demonstrates both the ferocity and compassion exhibited by the martial artist, like a hurricane compared to a gentle summer breeze. By the same token, the philosophy hidden in *Taegeuk Chil Jang,* with its image of the Mountain, teaches us when to take advantage of opportunity and when to pause, exercising caution and restraint in the process. Moreover, we can turn to *Taegeuk Pal Jang,* the last in the series, as a symbol of Earth or the Mother whose scrutiny concerning the growth and aptitude of her offspring is mirrored by the demands and complexity of the form itself. A great majority of the techniques the taekwondoist has been gifted with up to this point lie at the heart of poom-se Taegeuk Pal Jang and, like a mother checking for the correct number of toes and fingers on her newborn, constantly tests the practitioner's progress, sequence and technical focus.

After taking into account the essential role poom-se training plays in the development of traditional taekwondo technique, stamina, strength, focus, and defensive ability, we finally arrive at what may be its most profound intent. As indicated by this chapter's title, poom-se can be thought of as dynamic or moving meditation. This means that once the individual movements, rhythm, and mechanics of the form have been mastered, it can be performed almost without conscious thought. The martial artist's quest for enlightenment can then be realized by acting out or dwelling on the unique philosophical principles associated with the particular poom-se. The steps required in reaching this state of mind demand that the form first be learned on a purely physical level, making certain that each move becomes second nature. At this point the practitioner can begin to incorporate synchronized breathing, sequenced movement and hard/soft motions. Then and only then will the true philosophical value of the form begin to reveal itself in terms of meditative elegance. Obviously, this ability does not materialize overnight, but requires long hours of concentration and diligent practice. By working toward this goal, the true essence of poom-se training, outside the material realm, will clearly reveal itself to the taekwondo practitioner thus substantially adding to the spiritual rewards of the art.

Taekwondo poom-se are not only aesthetically pleasing to observe, but are also physically demanding and philosophically satisfying. Consequently, many practitioners are drawn to the martial arts based on their desire to master this form of dynamic meditation. Through poom-se practice, the body is strengthened and an acute sense of one's place in the universe is cultivated. Furthermore, since the foundation forms have been handed down from teacher to student over the years, they continue to act as stepping-stones on one's journey through the martial arts. Though inflections may differ somewhat from instructor to instructor, the major components have largely remained unchanged over time. This permanence adds to the traditional relevance of the forms and reminds us that while we are unique in our individual interpretation of taekwondo, we continue to be partners in the dynamically intensive, lethally effective, meditative dance we call poom-se.

CHAPTER 8

The Student/Teacher Relationship

Three centuries ago, seeking out a master and enrolling in a school of the martial arts was not as easy as it is today. Many times a potential student would be turned away based on their social standing or forced to wait an indeterminate amount of time prior to acceptance. Often, they would have to pass a test even before their application would be considered.

One such student, who after waiting two years to be admitted by the great Master Bukoden, discovered much to his dissatisfaction that his first lesson consisted of nothing more than working in the kitchen and stacking firewood. Six months later, discouraged and frustrated from carrying out these grueling chores, the student haltingly inquired as to when his formal sword training would truly begin. After not speaking to the student for much of their time together, the master stared into his eyes, declaring that lesson two would commence the following day. Late that night, as the student lay sleeping, the master crept silently into his room and began beating him with a *shinai* (bamboo sword.) Blow after blow rained down upon him as he attempted to protect himself. So started lesson two. From that day forward, it seemed every time the student would allow his defenses to drop, the master was suddenly there to attack, shinai in hand. This phase of his training continued for several years without further comment or explanation by the master. Soon, the student was permitted to carry a bamboo sword of his own, thus allowing him to clumsily parry his instructor's assaults. Try as he might, however, he could not avoid being beaten by Master Bukoden's well-aimed thrusts. As the months wore on, slowly and with great effort, the student's technique evolved to the point where he was able to draw his mock weapon in time to ward off the master's most severe attacks. Eventually, the student's awareness became so acute that his teacher could no longer strike him, even in the dead of night. Finally satisfied with his progress and proficiency, Master Bukoden broke his silence and demanded that his student meet with him the following morning. He was then presented with his diploma that consisted of a black ring painted on a rice paper background. This document, he was told, represented the mirror of his mind. Leaving his master, never to return, Miyamoto Musashi became Japan's greatest warrior. An undefeated swordsman, teacher, and samurai, he went on to author *The Book of Five Rings* in 1643—a volume widely read even to this day by martial artists and business people alike seeking strategic acumen.

The kinship that develops between a master and student of the martial arts is unlike any other that exists in everyday life. The depth of this alliance can fall anywhere between a passing acquaintance and prolonged discipleship. But what qualifications are necessary to become a master worthy of such intense devotion? In taekwondo, one must hold the rank of fourth dan black belt before being elevated to master status and seventh dan to become a grand master. Chronologically, this may take on the average of between ten to twenty years to achieve. However, time spent practicing the art is not the only indicator of one's ability to become a standard bearer of this Korean discipline. Attributes such as humility and understanding are essential since the candidate will be called upon to fill many roles. At times, the master instructor will act as counselor, confidant, spiritual advisor, parent figure, and in certain situations, a friend. He is the focal point, guide, and example of the student's martial arts training. So as not to take this bond too lightly, one must recall the foundation on which it is built. In spite of taekwondo's prominent philosophical components, the martial arts, by virtue of their definition, are based on a militaristic way of thinking. Seniority, discipline, rank, and decorum all come into play reflecting Asian cultural tradition as a whole. Therefore, as well as assuming the role of benefactor, the master instructor can at times appear tyrannical, demanding, and in extreme cases, masochistic. This potentially mercurial behavior is a direct result of the implied responsibilities that exist in the ever-evolving relationship between both the student and master.

It is important to note that for every obligation on the part of the instructor, there are obligations of equal importance on the part of the student. For example, critiquing a student's performance on a continuing basis is clearly part of the educational process and in no way should be construed as negative criticism. Likewise, it is the student's obligation to accept this criticism with gratitude and once identified, correct the deficiency in the most expedient way possible. Another shared obligation in the mutually expanding partnership between teacher and student is the development of trust. The master should feel confident that the student is sincere in his efforts while the practitioner needs to be assured that he is being offered the highest quality instruction available. Moreover, once a student has graduated to black belt, it then becomes his obligation to assist the instructor in teaching new students and helping out with the various administrative chores associated with dojang operations. Many Westerners cannot conceive of laboring in this manner without financial compensation. But as is the case with any journeyman connected to a guild or trade, one must learn through experience.

As indicated earlier, the martial arts are replete with an abundance of difficult techniques. A primary task of the instructor is to seek methods that will inspire and motivate the student to achieve goals far beyond those that they would normally think themselves capable of. While on the surface this may appear simple, it is not. Taekwondo classes are extremely challenging and many students find it difficult to unilaterally push themselves beyond their self-imposed limits. There have been endless instances where practitioners will insist on their inability to perform a particular kick or group of exercises only to discover, after the instructor applies the appropriate motivation, that the technique was well within their capabilities. It is here that the instructor's talents, acquired through years of experience, are revealed.

Furthermore, young and old alike will often seek advice regarding personal matters from their instructor. For many students, he or she is the one responsible for opening the door on a new and exciting way of life. Due to a pronounced spiritual connection, it is not uncommon for the practitioner to display a profound sense of devotion for their master. Taekwondo, being the empowering art that it is, instills values such as self-esteem

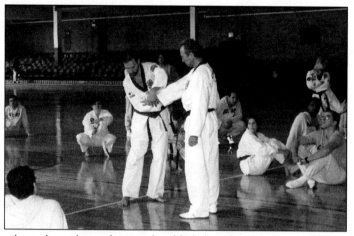

The taekwondo teacher is a humble link in the long chain of martial arts instruction. He or she must be sensitive not only to the students' physical needs, but to their spiritual and emotional requirements as well.

coupled with defensive skills that, in many cases, cannot be attained elsewhere. A truly competent instructor, therefore, is viewed by many as being on par with other professionals. Because of this, the instructor's advice and arbitration skill is naturally held in high regard. This situation presents a dilemma for many instructors truly concerned with their student's welfare. Should they question whether or not they should offer advice on topics in which they may or may not be qualified? Questions often come up on subjects pertaining to a child's performance in school, at home or in the dojang. Does the instructor answer based on an acquired knowledge of child psychology, or on the real-life experience gained from raising one's own offspring? Or, if an inquiry arises concerning ethics in the workplace, does the instructor respond through the eyes of a theologian or from the viewpoint of a guidance counselor? More appropriately, should advice be extended at all? Instructors are often faced with troubled individuals hoping to gain some insight or enlightenment as to the direction they should take in solving a personal problem. As we have seen, the measure of a true martial artist is not merely found in their sparring ability, but more in keeping with the holistic manner in which they approach life in general. Armed with the knowledge that students may solicit their advice, the conscientious instructor will act responsibly and speak from a position of strength having studied, albeit on an elementary level, the various topics to which they are most asked to respond. It is important to note however, that the master instructor is first and foremost a martial artist, and not a child psychologist or minister. It is purely at the instructor's discretion whether advice should be given or not. Refraining from offering advice should not be construed as a sign of incompetence but rather, in some cases, viewed as worthy advice in and of itself!

Since the instructor is often perceived as a purveyor of wisdom, is it any wonder then that many students are hard pressed to differentiate between their martial arts training and more traditional forms of academia? Certainly, when one considers the amount of time and diligence that is required in the pursuit of a martial discipline, a definite scholastic framework begins to emerge. Due to the similarities, there are those who equate their martial arts training with that of a full, matriculating college education. When viewed in this light, the role of the instructor begins to take on the overtones of a mentor or professor. This analogy is especially true given the Latin derivation of the word "education" which is, "to lead out." As the do in taekwondo signifies, the martial arts are a "way" or "path" through life and the master is there to guide and lead us. Being the senior partner, he or she must, at times, exercise the compassion and understanding of a father or mother with a child struggling to take its first steps. More than any other, this concept describes the ultimate function of the instructor. Within each of us lies the ability to perform a function at some level of proficiency. Certain individuals are athletically gifted and require little more than a brief demonstration before they are able to execute a particular technique with ease. By the same token, others require a great deal more attention and patience on the part of the teacher to become moderately proficient at the same technique. When accepting a student, therefore, the instructor assumes the implied responsibility of identifying the innate physical and mental qualities hidden within the student and cultivating these by whatever means necessary to ensure the success dictated by the chosen martial art. This does not give the teacher license to use excessive disciplinary measures as in the case of Miyamoto Musashi. Clearly, such actions as these would not be tolerated in today's society. However, as stated earlier, it is essential that the student realize his obligations. If the instructor is willing to give so freely of his or her hard earned knowledge, albeit for some financial remuneration, then certainly the student should reciprocate by training as hard and as diligently as possible. Subsequently, as an additional form of motivation, the instructor may choose to point out the practitioner's stronger techniques as well as those that may need work. A tried and true pedagogical tool that is found in the martial arts and can be applied to many similar situations in daily life, is a concept referred to as P/C/P or Praise/Correct/Praise. Before merely correcting an individual and running the risk of discouragement, an instructor will mention a positive performance, followed by the necessary criticism and conclude with yet another citation of the student's positive ability. This method allows the instructor to point out a

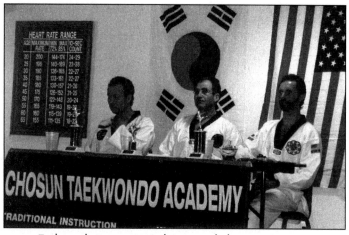

Taekwondo instructors judging at a belt promotion test.

student's weaknesses while simultaneously reinforcing his strengths.

Once again we are faced with a legitimate question: What value is there in the student/teacher relationship, and how does it affect the way we pattern our lives on a daily basis? In today's world, many of the relationships we build, whether they are of a marital, social, or familial nature, are often permitted to deteriorate to the point of dissolution based primarily on our inability to cope with an ever-changing emotional landscape. This malady is further exacerbated by the many distractions we are faced with moment by moment. Broadcast history shows that television scenes change much more rapidly today than in the past, largely due to a decrease in the viewer's overall attention span. In a scholastic setting, our children are routinely marched from room to room, teacher to teacher, year after year, never to anchor on a single instructor's personality. Our friendships, in many cases, are brought to an abrupt halt attributed to some minor disagreement that is forgotten about the following day in part because we do not take the time to analyze the situation before losing control. Marriages and families are split because we find difficulty expressing the compassion and tenacity

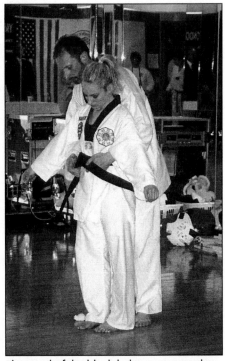

The ritual of the black belt ceremony echoes the union found in marriage.

we so much desire for ourselves. Who do we blame for these deficiencies in our character? Parents? Teachers? Before remedial action can be taken, the symptom must first be identified. In the majority of cases the symptom is a broken or damaged relationship. The problem, clearly, is a lack of patience or training in maintaining a prolonged relationship. As with other scenarios in life, it is much easier simply to walk away from a difficult partnership rather than to stay and work things out. The martial arts offer viable solutions to these problems in the form of required attendance, respect for instructors, seniors and peers, and the inculcation of confidence in oneself. As a case in point, sometime during the enrollment orientation, most instructors will notify a youngster's parents concerning the importance of regularly attending class on a set schedule. Left to their own designs, the student who manufacturers excuses for missing class, whether it be due to a feigned illness or a bout of laziness, will fall into a vicious cycle of absenteeism that will eventually infest other portions of the practitioner's life. Consequently, the novice student should be encouraged at all costs to attend class even in the face of real or imagined adversity. This facet of the child's training cannot be over-emphasized, for it is here that the foundation for future alliances is laid. Clearly, the above is equally true for the adult practitioner as well. More importantly, however, if taken seriously and allowed to mature, the student/teacher relationship offers an identifiable consistency in the shape of a paternal-like bond not found in other

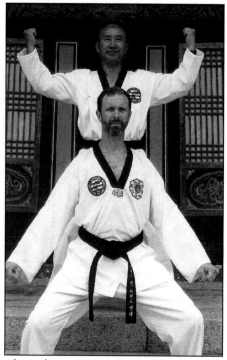

The author, Kyosanim Doug Cook, with his instructor, Grand Master Richard Chun, practicing at Pulguksa temple in Korea.

areas. For example, during the black belt ceremony, an observer will notice that the instructor symbolically bestows the student with a portion of his wisdom by first wrapping the belt around his waist before tying it around the student's. Even though the student may, in the future, train with other instructors, this is a statement that clearly says, "I am your only true master and you are tied to me for now and forever." This ritual is vaguely reminiscent of another, equally heavy with meaning—that found in the bond of marriage. Once a serious commitment is made to a study of the martial arts, one cannot simply ignore its implications.

Regardless of title, whether it is Sensei, Sabumnim,

Kyosanim, or Sifu, the instructor holds the future to the practitioner's martial life, quite literally, in his hands. His students are living reflections of the virtues he exemplifies. They echo his physical technique as well as the philosophical and spiritual values he espouses. Through strength he teaches discipline; through humility, compassion; through encouragement, self-esteem. He shares a common bond with the teachers of the past. In the end though, the instructor has the awesome responsibility of passing on a martial tradition that he has personally refined in some small way, thus leaving his mark for the future generations of martial artists to come.

CHAPTER 9

With Total Commitment

Prior to becoming involved in the martial arts, it is difficult for the untrained person to visualize some of the more elusive benefits taekwondo has to offer. While sparring and breaking are two of the more dramatic physical manifestations of the art, hidden beneath the surface lie other truly valuable attributes. In previous chapters we touched on Asian philosophy, martial doctrine, and ancient history. It is now time to examine some of the less obvious but equally fundamental underpinnings of taekwondo—that of extreme focus, determination, and will. These characteristics constitute the necessary ingredients to execute martial technique and daily living with total commitment.

Focus in the martial arts can be defined as the consolidation of one's internal energy funneled and projected upon a given target. Our target does not necessarily need to be of a tangible nature such as a kicking pad or focus mitt—it can just as easily be represented by a real life situation. In order to attain maximum focus, however, concentration is essential in that the body and mind must be unified. If full results are expected from a technique, the practitioner needs to maintain a steady stream of awareness, for if the mind is wandering, the body is weak. Strength, power, and speed amount to nothing without concentration. According to Koichi Tohei, founder of Shin Shin Toitsu Aikido or "Aikido with Mind and Body Coordinated," both aspects must be brought together similar to the manner in which two front wheels of an automobile are required to turn in tandem if the vehicle is to arrive at its proper destination. But, Sang Kyu Shim may have put it best in his work, *The Making of A Martial Artist,* when he said, "When an individual converts concentration into action, the movement is called focus. A vitalized mental image becomes a physical reality. The combination of concentration and focus intensifies power two, four, tenfold."

The quintessence of determination is thought of as the act of deciding a matter definitely and firmly. Essentially, there are three stages in determination. Firstly, recognizing a decision needs to be made or a situation acted upon. Secondly, arriving at a solution in a logical and thoughtful fashion and lastly, resolutely acting upon it. Once a decision is made, therefore, one should then carry it through, content in the knowledge that a solution has been arrived at. Taekwondo is an action philosophy. What we mean by this is that its pursuit adds vibrancy to one's life. It imbues the practitioner with the self-confidence it takes to make and then stand behind difficult decisions precisely as a modern day warrior should. This does not infer inflexibility, however. Standing behind a decision even though it has created an injustice is a travesty of the modern day martial arts ideal. Along with confidence, then, one should also exhibit the courage to reverse such a decision if it appears the prudent thing to do.

Defining the will, on the other hand, is another matter entirely. This evanescent entity, it is believed, will in certain situations of life or death ultimately determine if we survive. Many times we hear of an individual "losing the will to live" or of "having the will to go on." Our will is the partner that sits us up in bed in the morning, plants our feet firmly on the floor and prepares us for the day ahead. Clearly, if one loses will, the ability to live life to its fullest potential is also lost. Will is something that cannot be taught but acts as the spark or catalyst that stokes the fires of our determination. Whether it be breaking a patio block with a hammer fist (*me chumok*), or the decision to begin a new business venture, once determination has been firmly established by the will, we can then focus on the matter at hand. A magical synergy begins to evolve—the sum of which is equal to more than its parts.

Il Kyuk Pil Sul is a Korean creed that is sometimes recited during the closing ritual of a class. Translated into English as "first strike, swift and complete," these few short syllables clearly reflect the essence of commitment as it pertains to taekwondo. Were we to ever be physically threatened and forced to put our defensive skills to the test, these movements would need to be executed with total commitment. It is the belief, especially in the Korean martial arts, that the initial blow should be all that is required to immobilize an opponent. Hesitation or reluctance in combat can mean injury or death. One may not be given a second opportunity to act. The techniques we learn cannot and will not be effective unless the dynamics of will, determination, focus, and commitment are instantly applied. As in the preparation of a tasty stew, the lack of a key ingredient will be noticed. The same holds true for the four attributes above; one cannot exist without the other in the martial arts.

Moreover, each day of our life it seems we are faced with tasks both large and small, difficult or routine. Given the choice we can either shy away from these tasks or attack them head on. Upon closer examination, we find that this principle lies at the heart of taekwondo training. When our instructor presents the gift of a new technique to us, what is our response? Do we embrace it with the determination, will, focus and commitment necessary to master it, or do we cheat ourselves and shrink away from the challenge? Clearly, one of the many goals of the martial arts is to achieve the highest level of proficiency our belt level allows. This is only possible, however, if we approach each new lesson with determination and execute it to the best of our ability.

Consider for a moment the fact that many of the Asian empty-hand fighting arts were developed for a people generally smaller in physical stature than their Western or European counterparts. If strength alone were the determining factor in the successful application of these martial disciplines, then perhaps there would be considerably less sovereign territory today in Japan or Korea given the long, bloody history of war and occupation they both have in common. Since the early days of the Koguryo kingdom, Korea alone has been occupied by invading forces on more than nine hundred separate occasions. Furthermore, when we take into account the gallantry and valor displayed by the Hwarang, coupled with the courage of Japan's samurai class and compare that spirit with the astonishing business and cultural revivals shared by these nations since World War II and the Korean conflict, we see further evidence that the "Budo" or warrior instinct has not only survived, but continues to flourish. It is this emphasis on living and working with total commitment that has stimulated and maintained this remarkable resurgence.

By now it should be apparent that by accepting advancement, we are simultaneously accepting the inherent responsibilities that come with each new belt level. The cloak of competency we proudly wear, however, requires that we set a worthy example for our juniors. In the martial arts, as in most hierarchies, lower belts continuously look up to their seniors for direction. Therefore, training with total commitment on a purely physical level is one way an example can best be set. Once, while attending a Taekwondo training camp, I had the experience of putting this concept into practice. With the participating students ranging from four to sixty years of age, the camp was held in a particularly tranquil setting in upper New York State. The foothills of the Catskill Mountains offered an environment that lent itself to quiet meditation and uninterrupted physical training. Although unseasonably warm and humid, the June weather promised not a hint of rain. On the first evening of our arrival, we quickly stowed our packs in our assigned cabins beneath the trees and were called together to meditate on the shore of a lake dotted on its surface with the activity of the wildlife below. But it was on the second day that our training began in earnest. Following a light breakfast and a brief period of meditation to prepare our minds for what lay ahead, we jogged through the woods single file until we reached a wide, open meadow bordered by the lake on one side and a swift running brook on the other. Being the senior black belt in attendance, I brought the students to attention, bowed and awaited further instructions. The head instructor commanded us to begin by stepping forward with basic stances, blocks and strikes. This continued for approximately an hour as the morning sun began to peek over the tops of the trees. Already we became aware of the rising temperature as the perspiration began to soak through our doboks. Taking full advantage of deep breathing techniques, our bodies were replenished with a healthy supply of fresh oxygen as the morning session continued with a series of kicking drills and flexibility training. Even though the advanced techniques were difficult, a sense of elation prevailed. Shortly, however, a look of exhaustion could be detected on the faces of the participants as the noon break approached. After lunch and a brief rest, we returned to our "dojang under the sky" and prepared for the afternoon session.

During poom-se practice, a combination of the hot afternoon sun and the food we had just eaten began to take its toll and our fatigue quickly became apparent. I found my mind wandering and as a result, made several foolish errors during my execution of the form Taegeuk Sam Jang. Slowly, visions of the Hwarang training began to creep into my consciousness. Willing myself back to the moment, I refocused; forgetting the aches in my body and with each strike projected my ki energy with renewed vigor. Those around me seemed to sense the revitalization in my voice as my kihop echoed across the field. The energy began to ripple outward until a chorus of spirit yells could be heard rebounding off the surrounding hills. Moving in almost perfect unison, we continued with our poom-se, this time performing each movement with total commitment. The remainder of the afternoon, filled with yoga, calisthenics, self-defense techniques and endurance drills, passed quickly. Talking later, it seemed we had all experienced a similar feeling of invigoration in spite of the intense training and the heat of the afternoon. This is but a humble illustration of what the will in combination with focus and a totally committed mind can achieve under relatively extreme circumstances.

As a personal form of expression, taekwondo is an ever-evolving art. It is not enough to simply visit the training hall once or twice a week only to leave what we have learned beside the door of the changing rooms. We must, instead, constantly grow, taking these lessons and applying them in a practical man-

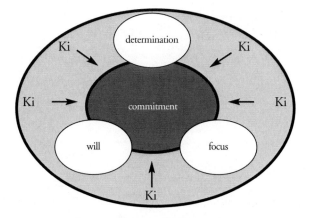

The Components of Commitment.

ner to whatever our life demands at any given moment. Therefore, training with total commitment means not only putting everything you can into your physical technique, but also grasping every opportunity that is offered to you. This may mean putting fear of failure aside if the specter of change presents itself, or keeping discouragement at bay should the tide of events turn against you. Even though we attempt to plan for the future, we can never be truly certain what our daily routine may hold. It is of the utmost importance, therefore, to maintain concentration and awareness while relying on a strong will, a determined mind, and sharp focus. It is the sum of these virtues that can often make the difference between long-term success or tragic failure. Consequently, whether you are a surgeon cutting human tissue or a jeweler cutting diamonds, a carpenter driving nails or a trucker driving an eighteen-wheeler, in order to accomplish any endeavor correctly the modern day warrior must approach the job with total commitment.

CHAPTER 10

Ki: The Universal Life Force

Central to any study of Western medicine and the associated life sciences is a deep understanding of the various elements that go into making up the human body. Medical students are taught early on about the biosystems that transport blood to the cells, oxygen from the lungs, and nerve impulses to the brain. But their professors reveal little, if anything, regarding the mysterious system of meridians and acupoints that run throughout the body. This system is thought to channel the vital life force known in the Korean and Japanese cultures as *ki* and to the Chinese as *qi* or *chi*. First mention of qi theory can be traced back to the birth of Traditional Chinese Medicine during the reign of the Yellow Emperor, Huang Di (2697-2597 B.C.). It was during this period that Huang Di authored the *Nei Jing Su Wen,* or *Classic on Internal Medicine,* that remains the basis for Chinese medical practice to this day.

In his exceptional volume, *Ki: A Practical Guide for Westerners*, William Reed, a disciple of Koichi Tohei, defines ki as, "A universal energy, capable of infinite expansion and contraction, which can be directed, but not contained by the mind." Master Fa Xiang Hou of the Qigong Research Society contends that, "Qi flows through all living things, circulating among the organs, and is comprised of both Yin and Yang forces." In noting the universal nature of the vital life force, Grand Master Richard Chun, a worldwide pioneer and practitioner of traditional taekwondo states, "Ki is the cosmic ocean in which everything exists." These explanations, though oddly similar to those found in modern Christianity when describing the human soul, may appear somewhat metaphysical in nature to the ears of the Occidental. In spite of this, there are those in the West who have become intimately familiar with qi through the practice of the Chinese discipline taijiquan. It is reputed that Zhang, San-Feng developed the principles on Wudang Mountain located to the south of Hubei Province in China during the Song dynasty (960-1280 A.D.). By performing a series of long and short patterns, similar to taekwondo poom-se or karate kata, practitioners of this demanding Taoist style strive to manipulate the flow of what essentially can be referred to as the essence of life. Aikido, the popular Japanese martial art derived from daito-ryu akijujutsu, also encourages strong ki development since its main emphasis is on blending with an opponent's attack, thus effectively turning the aggressor's negative ki against him. On a more therapeutic level, the widespread acceptance of acupuncture as a supplement to conventional medical procedures, has lent additional credibility to the ki-bearing meridial system. By the well-placed insertion of needles, the acupuncturist treats illness by effecting the various acupoints stationed throughout the body.

Ki development can have a beneficial effect on those from all walks of life. Clearly, martial artists, as such, do not hold a monopoly on the vital life force or its refinement. Ki flows through all living things—from the microscopic, single-celled amoebas, to the most glorious and complex life form of all, the human being. Unlike the circulatory, respiratory or nervous systems, definitive evidence of ki has yet to be satisfactorily established in the laboratory. Since clinical data is currently unavailable confirming this elusive system, how can we be certain it positively exists? Because we are largely a people who require tangible proof of a concept before we can commit to its existence, efforts continue on the part of researchers to measure the presence of ki. Although currents closely following the body's internal network of meridians have been electronically detected and human auras surrounding the body captured on film, skepticism of this bioelectric system prevails.

Practitioners of Traditional Chinese Medicine (TCM) have been treating patients for centuries by manipulating the action of the ki system through the use of herbs, acupuncture, and deep massage. While physicians in the West have historically relied on medication to remedy illness, Eastern medical doctrine has chosen instead to avoid sickness by maintaining a correct balance of the vital life force within the body. The importance of this statement becomes abundantly clear when one accepts the fact that pain and illness occurs as a function of ki blockages or imbalances. Knowing this, ki equilibrium can be achieved in a variety of ways. Of the several methods available, including meditation and deep breathing, qigong exercise and therapy is at the forefront. Over three thousand years old, qigong practice promotes health and longevity through the performance of a series of exercises geared towards providing the practitioner with an innate sense of well being and physical fitness. Under the guidance of an accomplished qigong master, the practitioner learns to move, circulate, and manipulate ki energy throughout the entire body over a series of channels or meridians. In addition, qigong therapy utilizes bodywork, acupuncture, and herbal medicines to stimulate a healthy flow of ki. These methods ultimately result in a more responsive immune system and overall good health, Many qigong masters live past the age of one hundred. In an article for *Black Belt* magazine titled, "Milestones in the Chinese Martial Arts," writer Jane Hallander states, "Qigong itself is not a martial art. It is a Chinese internal regimen used to improve health, develop better breathing patterns, and strengthen a person's internal ki power. Qigong practice directly relates to the quality of a person's martial arts ability. Thanks to the immigration and visits of numerous Chinese qigong experts, American martial artists are able to combine qigong practice with their fighting arts practice, therefore developing martial arts expertise that rivals practitioners anywhere else in the world."

Explaining the presence and movement of ki can often prove

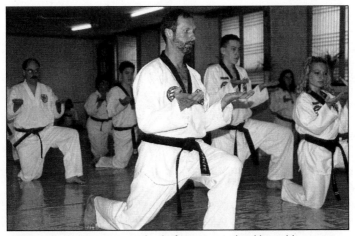

Qigong Exercise is a method of promoting health and longevity while balancing the body's ki energy.

confusing to the Western mind. In an effort to explain this circulation, we must compare ki theory to anatomical systems we are more familiar with. For instance, when we are cut, blood flows from the wound and can be physically touched and seen. Ki energy cannot be handled, but, like the wind, can be felt and observed. It is similar to the light emanating from a movie projector. Even though one cannot hold the individual photons or quanta of energy in their hands, the resultant image can be viewed on the screen. So it is with ki. Like the projector, it radiates outward originating from the midsection, approximately two inches below the navel. Known in Korean as the tjan tjin, Japanese as *tanden,* and Chinese as the *dantian,* this area is thought to be the internal reservoir where ki is stored. Similarly, the tjan tjin can be viewed as the center of one's internal universe or as a furnace generating untold quantities of energy. According to Reed, the tjan tjin is also referred to as the one point and can alternatively be described as "a tiny star or vortex sucking in immense amounts of energy from the universe." From this center, the vital life force travels through two main vessels running up the front and back of the body, eventually reaching the internal organs and extremities through twelve additional meridians branching off into pairs. These channels can be likened to a railroad line with the stations being the pressure or accupoints. Ki travels along the track, as would a train delivering energy to the various points along the way. Should any of these channels become clogged, the ki flow will become inhibited and illness will result. The purpose of ki development is to keep these meridians clear of blockages, thus encouraging an unobstructed, healthy flow of ki. How then does ki enter and reach the tjan tjin in the first place?

Since ki energy is universal and airborne, our body's primary source is through the air we breathe. Correct breathing, therefore, is essential to proper ki development. Breathing, being an unconscious, involuntary reflex, naturally leads many of us to assume we are performing it correctly. In most cases, however, quite the converse is true. In all likelihood, the last person to coach us in correct breathing was the physician who delivered us from the womb. The time worn practice of striking an infant on the buttocks at birth causes it to gulp in great quantities of life-sustaining air. This air does not merely settle in the lungs, but is taken down deep into the area of the diaphragm. Weeks later, if one were to observe the same infant lying in its crib, he would notice the rhythmic rise and fall of its abdominal region with each passing breath. This is because, rather than taking light, measured breaths, it continues to take long, deep inhalations, and exhalations culminating in the tjan tjin. For whatever reason though, as we age our body forgets to breathe in this fashion. As we mature, we begin to trade deep, ki-enriched breathing for that of the short, shallow variety. This is truly unfortunate since there is a direct correlation among the integrity of the individual organs, blood circulation and deep breathing. Blood completes a full circuit of the body, delivering nutrients and oxygen it receives from the air we breath in a surprisingly short period of time. In order to satisfy the demands of every living cell, the blood relies on the respiratory system to replenish it with a fresh supply of oxygen and ki. It is a fact that strong, healthy cells can become maligned if a proper level of oxygen is not maintained. In addition, waste products must be removed with help from the lymphatic system. Correct breathing allows the blood to become saturated with oxygen upon inhalation while, during exhalation, aids in eliminating unwanted metabolic byproducts. By taking advantage of deep breathing, therefore, the dual requirements of ki delivery and cleansing will be satisfied.

Being aware of the significant role correct breathing plays in maintaining a healthy body, we must now ask how this tool can be used by the martial artist to augment technique. When the student learns to utilize proper breathing as a strategic weapon, he will come to realize that the prime moment to attack is when the opponent is inhaling rather than exhaling. This is when the adversary is most vulnerable since the muscles offer the least protection to the skeletal structure and internal organs when they are in a flaccid and relaxed state. In contrast, exhaling will produce the opposite effect by adding ki power to an attack and pulling the body's musculature taut as required in a defensive posture. The sports-minded will find deep, controlled breathing essential when competing since endurance is directly proportional to our ki/oxygen intake. Controlled breathing also aids in masking exhaustion during sparring (kyoreugi). Gasping for breath shows an opponent that they may have already gained the winning edge.

So far we have seen the benefits of qigong practice and correct breathing on ki development. Let us now examine yet another method used in cultivating the universal life force—meditation. Meditation, as we shall see, assumes many roles in the practice of the martial arts. In the case of ki development meditation is used to attract, visualize, intensify, and manipulate the vital life force within the body. One simple, yet effective method is used at the beginning of selected training sessions in order to revitalize the student's ki energy. Finding a comfortable location, the practitioner sits in a lotus position, legs crossed, one upon the other. If this is not possible, a half lotus position is acceptable. The back must be straight with the nose in line with the navel. The hands are placed on the knees with the palms open and facing up. Hand positioning is important because a critical ki receptor, the laogong, is located in the center of the palm. Likewise, as dictated by many Eastern cultures, the upper dantian or "third eye," is found in the middle of the forehead. This area is also sensitive to ki reception. While inhaling deeply, the person meditating closes their eyes and visualizes a bright point in space sending forth an intense stream of ki. Imagining the upper dantian opening and acting as a gateway, the universal energy continues to flow downward through the main meridian as it fills the dantian or tjan tjin. By touching the tip of the tongue to the roof of the mouth, a link or connection is made between the two main vessels that run through the front and rear of the body. The saliva that accumulates should be swallowed thus keeping the throat moist. Exhaling, the visualization continues with ki leaving the dantian, climbing up the meridial system, and streaming out the upper dantian. To avoid confusion, it must be remembered that the dantian, tanden, and tjan tjin are synonymous depending on the culture from which the term originates. After practicing this meditation for a time, the dantian and laogong may grow warm or begin to tingle and can be taken as an indicator of active ki circulation.

The concept of ki and its manipulation is a common thread that runs through the philosophical fabric shared by many martial disciplines. Korean history alone, for example, is overflowing with

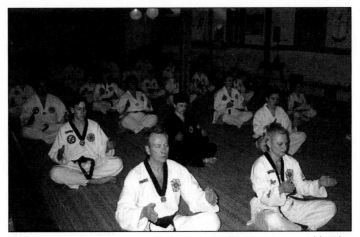

Taekwondo students cultivate ki through meditation. Ki is used by the martial artist to amplify technique.

heroic figures performing inconceivable feats of valor stemming from a ki-laden will. Today, tales of magic abound with stories of mothers single-handedly lifting the full weight of an automobile in order to free a child pinned beneath or, in the case of the taekwondoist, the demonstration of seemingly miraculous breaking techniques and dramatic flying kicks. It is not unheard of, therefore, for members of the general public to ascribe mystical powers or superhuman strength to the martial artist. While their basic assumption may stray shy of the mark, the observation hinting at some form of hidden power is credible. Unbeknownst to the average person, what they are attempting to describe is the practitioner's ability to extend and direct ki. We do not simply mean reaching the hand or foot further out into space while punching or kicking. Instead, ki should be thought of as a laser beam reaching to the far ends of the cosmos, boring its way through the target and making a strong and unbreakable connection between its eventual destination and the practitioner's tjan tjin or one point. Furthermore, ki projection does not need to originate solely from a fist or foot, but can alternately be emitted in the form of a kihop, issuing from the tjan tjin. This shout not only has the ability to initially startle an opponent, breaking his concentration, but also saturates the body and the immediate area with ki energy. However, it is essential to bear in mind that the report of a pistol is meaningless if it is exclusively loaded with blank rounds.

Likewise, speed, power and proper technique must accompany the kihop in order to be successful. On the other hand, the accomplished martial artist learns to apply controlled pressure to the numerous cavities or acupoints found at various locations on the body. The manipulation of these pressure points can be used either to inflict great pain or restore health as in the case of acupressure.

If in truth there are any *okuden* or "secret techniques" buried in the conventional model of the martial arts, they are rooted in the virtues of ki development accompanied by vigorous training, deep breathing, and meditation. Through the cultivation of strong ki, the taekwondoist in particular can develop technique that is focused, fluid, effective and at the same time, acutely sensitive to surrounding circumstances. Consequently, it is within the domain of the modern day warrior to uncover the hidden ways of developing and using ki to its greatest advantage both inside and outside the dojang. Moreover, the science of physics teaches us that energy can be altered but not destroyed. In the martial arts we see the manifestation of this principle in the duality of opposites and the ever-circulating flow of ki. Balanced ki is what separates the martial artist from the pugilist, the healthy from the sick, the living from the dead. Furthermore, by exuding positive ki as we walk our daily path, we affect others within our sphere of influence, thus allowing them to share in a more wholesome life experience as well. And what better way is there for the practitioner to set an appropriate example? Therefore, it is the goal, indeed the mandate, of every martial artist, to utilize the tools of proper ki development in maintaining a balanced and harmonious relationship with nature and in the end, the Universe as a whole.

The Benefits of Meditation

Since the beginning of time, mankind has attempted to push
back the veil of ignorance in search of wisdom and power. As
a matter of survival, enemies that could be seen were quickly
vanquished through the use of physical force and strategic
thinking. However, adversaries of pure thought, those lurking in
the mind, were more difficult to identify and overcome. Even
though over the centuries we as a people have learned to master
advanced forms of technology, our quest for enlightenment has
not yet been satisfied and continues to this day with equal, if
not accelerated, vigor. Why has contentment of the spirit not
run parallel to our acquisition of knowledge? Many would contend that as the human race moves closer to controlling its des-
tiny through technology and modern science, we are moving
further from finding true inner peace. We are trading our connection with a world of intangible, yet vastly superior values, for
those of instant, short term, gratification. How can we regain
some of the high ground we have surrendered in our lust for
material wealth?

To the uninitiated, the practice of meditation denotes, in its
most benign sense, a form of relaxation. To skeptical others, the
thought of emptying the brain of unbridled thought conjures up
images of mystics and mind-manipulating demons. In truth, the
act of meditation caters to a common need to recover a portion
of our consciousness that has been blunted by everyday life in a
highly technical society. It serves as a conduit to self-realization
and a means of quieting the restless winds that blow through our
minds. Broadly speaking, sitting in quiet reflection provides a
tool that allows us to gain control of our body and spirit.
Meditation can be thought of as a crew of workers that constantly maintains the bridge between mind and body since, as we
now know, internal development must occur simultaneous with
physical development in the martial arts. Taijiquan master

Herman Kauz observes in his book, *The Martial Spirit*, that, "becoming aware of how we think and feel about ourselves is perhaps the first and most important step in changing our lives for the better."

It is significant to note that students beginning the martial arts do so for many reasons other than the spiritual and may find it difficult to understand why meditation plays such a pre-dominant role. A great majority are drawn by the desire to learn a form of self-defense as a means of protection while others may view their training as a way to attain a heightened state of physical fitness. In addition, along with the parent looking to enter their child in a competitive sport, there are also those seeking discipline, self-esteem or social interaction. The passage of time, however, has a tendency to affect these motives, causing them to assume an air of superficiality. A serious student eventually comes to the realization that there exists a deeper meaning to their study of the martial arts. Thus, the practice of meditation also acts as a key, unlocking a door to these sensitivities.

As it applies to the art of taekwondo, the practice of meditation has many faces. First and foremost, it is traditionally used during the opening ritual to clear the mind prior to beginning class. Why is this necessary? Regardless of whether the student is an adult frustrated by the affairs of the day, or a youngster concerned about schoolwork, it is not uncommon to enter the dojang burdened by excess mental baggage. Any stray thoughts that may inhibit concentration must be eliminated in order to make room for the lessons at hand. Once again, acting metaphorically as a bridge, meditation gently carries us from one reality to another. At the command of "Muk Yum" (meditation), this essential portion of the curriculum is accomplished by sitting quietly in a lotus or half lotus position with hands turned, palms facing up and placed on the knees. Breathing deeply with eyes closed, we can virtually feel the tension drain from the body. Meditation, like an eraser, wipes a blackboard clean. It clears the mind and allows it to accept fresh ideas. Likewise, at the completion of class, it is helpful to utilize this method in reverse while reflecting on the various techniques we have learned. By replaying the movements in our mind shortly after their execution, they become ingrained and easier to recall at a later date during our own personal practice. This is similar to reading a book more than once—we may retain segments of the text missed the first or second time through and savor them in a different light. Clearly, this form of meditation, used to relax and retain information, can be put into practice in any number of ways during our daily life.

Secondly, meditation can be thought of as a forum for contemplation—a mental stage that allows the practitioner to visualize a particular facet of training or philosophy. In a meditative state, the mind can be more responsive to visualization. Since the body follows the mind, this form of internal focus can be used to coax thoughts into becoming reality. An example of this can be found in the Olympic champion who, when asked, attributes at least a modicum of his success to visualizing or seeing a perfect performance through the mind's eye days or even weeks prior to the actual event. As one would imagine, meditative visualization can prove helpful in a variety of situations as it pertains to the martial artist.

Traditionally, belt promotion tests have been a source of great anxiety to the novice. By putting this visual technique into effect during meditation, the student can virtually assure his success through suggestive measures, thus mirroring the Olympian. A student who is expecting to test for promotion should first be mentally prepared. By visualizing the examination, including waking up the morning of the test after getting plenty of sleep, having a nutritious breakfast, and knowing ahead of time that his uniform and all necessary equipment is packed and ready to go, the student will already have gained a significant advantage. By frequently following through on this exercise, the practitioner can see the events that lay ahead unfold in their mind. This will ultimately prove less stressful because they have cognitively "been there" and have already passed the test. The image flows forward in time, as the practitioner visualizes driving to the dojang, walking in to discover a crowd of spectators, then stretching out and meditating after changing into his dobok. At this point the student can almost hear his name being called and running up to the required position to begin the test. He is confident of success, knowing he is ready. The instructor would not permit him to be there if he were not. After much anticipation,

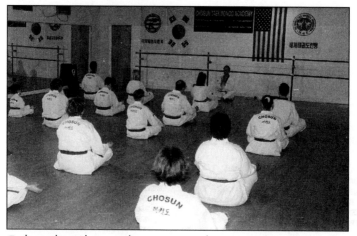

Taekwondo students meditating prior to beginning class. The mind is calmed in preparation for the lessons to come.

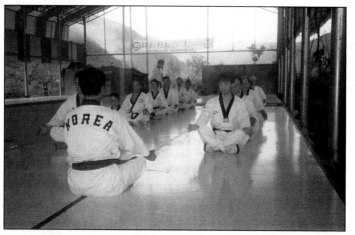

Practicing Zen meditation in Da Han village, Korea.

the test finally begins and all that the practitioner has visualized begins to unfold. The expected nervousness sets in but is quickly replaced by the confidence and knowledge that he will do his best. With a clear and relaxed mind, the candidate begins the test. Hours later, the instructor is wrapping the hard-earned belt around his waist while he basks in the glow of satisfaction and relief. On the surface, this method may appear somewhat simplistic, but it will cause the student to relax and gain confidence at the same time.

Meditative visualization, as it is described above, may erroneously cause one to conclude that anything from daydreaming to worry can be meditation. But, unlike these two common preoccupations that thrive on scattered thought, meditation can act as a lens focusing the mind on a single thought and, eventually, no thought at all. In what may first appear to be a paradox, the ability to achieve this highly concentrated state of consciousness despite the violent action associated with martial arts, lies at the core of Eastern theology. During the late fifth century when Bodhidharma began teaching his style of gongfu to the monks of the Shaolin temple, ethical doctrines unique to Asian religious philosophy began to merge with physical techniques common to the martial arts. Since the spiritual requirements of both seemed consistent with one another, this union appeared inevitable. In a practical sense, these early Asian fighting skills taught by the Zen patriarch were employed as protection against roving bandits and spiritually strengthened the body in preparation for advanced forms of physically demanding meditation. However, the fact that certain religious sects or leaders of distinction chose to blend, create or become proficient in a particular defensive style, is of secondary importance. What is important is an appreciation of the impact these various religious influences would have on the evolution of the martial arts. For example, on the wings of Taoism came proper breathing techniques coupled with the doctrine of non-intervention as exemplified in modern aikido. Likewise, the Korean nobility borrowed heavily from Confucianism, using it as a moral compass in the formulation of the Hwarang-do ethical standards. Then, as today, both philosophical viewpoints are of paramount importance to the martial artist.

Most notable, however, is the contribution made by Zen (Sun in Korean) Buddhism as it relates to *zazen,* a seated style of meditation developed by Dogen, a Zen monk in the year 1253. The goal of zazen, as it is practiced by Zen's Soto sect, is to reach a state of *satori* or "enlightenment" by releasing the mind from all random thought until conscious recognition of the physical realm is replaced by spiritual harmony with all that is. This ultimately leads to a deep appreciation of the moment rather than cluttering the intellect with concerns of the past or future.

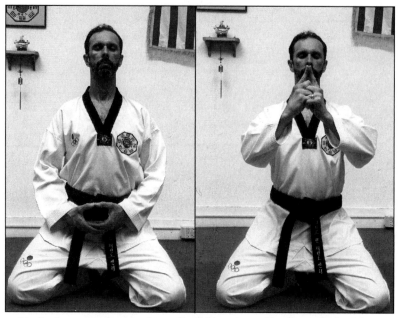

Meditation using the cosmic mudra (left) and mind-body mudra (right). A mudra is a hand gesture used during meditation to achieve that which is symbolized and to seal in ki energy.

Historically, meditation of this sort has played a vital role in the warrior's ability to survive. In ancient times, the seconds required for conscious thought before delivering a blow in battle would surely have resulted in certain injury or even death. Without a doubt, the advantages provided to the samurai by mental preparation through meditation quickly became apparent. Furthermore, the religious beliefs espoused by Zen Buddhism dovetailed with the warriors code of honor in that at any time they may be called upon to forfeit their lives for king and country while walking the razor's edge between spiritual strength and physical reality.

Warfare notwithstanding, modern artistic technique also demands rapid reaction time. For, unlike modern sport where a failed pass or missed swing is acceptable, there is no room in the martial arts for hesitation. This principle requires the martial artist to develop a form of meditation-in-motion referred to by the Japanese as *mushin* or "mind/no-mind." Once attained, the practitioner can move from stance to stance, unhindered by the thought process, thus allowing him to react instantly, naturally, and efficiently. Subsequently, zazen continues to be used by the Zen master in search of enlightenment as well as the martial artist preparing the mind for immediate action. Eventually, being acutely sensitive to his surroundings as well as totally engrossed in the moment, the practitioner can defend against a technique even before his opponent has had an opportunity to pounce. Clearly, this talent may require years of training coupled with concentrated sessions of Zen meditation to achieve.

Learning zazen meditation requires patience and effort on the part of the modern day warrior. In essence, our mind can be compared to an unbroken stallion galloping wildly and without direction until brought under control by a competent trainer. Similarly, we must learn to distill our shifting thoughts down to a single, focused point. Since this is an acquired skill and not a born talent, we must take advantage of the resources made available through Zen practice. These include the use of koans, mudras, mantras, and breath counting. A *koan* is a riddle with no apparent logical answer used in hopes of exhausting the mind into a state of release or satori. An example of a koan can be, "What is the sound of one hand clapping?" Conversely, a *mudra* is a hand gesture assumed in a meditation posture that has the ability to achieve what it symbolizes. Use

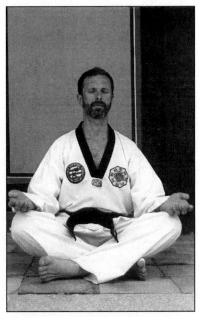

The author meditating at Puluksa temple in Korea. The open palms act as a receptor for ki energy.

of a mudra can have a surprisingly dramatic effect on one's ability to consolidate thought. In order to soothe the brain, one may rely on the use of a *mantra*. This is a phrase or word repeated again and again which will eventually be lost during the meditative process, leaving the mind in a state of solitude. Westerners may be familiar with the mantra syllable "Om" which is often used. The novice practitioner may discover breath counting to be the simplest and most direct approach. To begin, one must assume the correct posture. This is accomplished by sitting in a lotus position, legs crossed with ankles drawn up into the lap. The back must be straight with the nose remaining in line with the navel. The eyes should be closed or partially open as long as it is not distracting. The recommended mudra for zazen meditation is one where the back of one hand is placed in the palm of the other. The thumbs then touch one another thus forming an oval that is placed in the lap resting on the abdomen two inches below the navel. This is known as the cosmic mudra and is meant to aid in attracting and centering ki energy. Once the above requirements have been met, we are then prepared to begin proper breathing techniques. At this point we start by counting our exhalations only. Taking a deep breath in through the nose, we hold it for a moment, pushing it down to the tjan tjin or diaphragm area. Upon exhalation, which lasts a bit longer

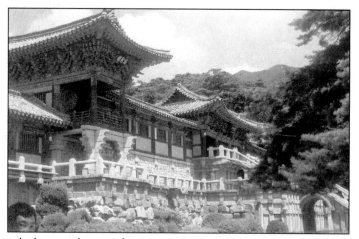

Pulguksa temple in southeast Korea is a monument to both the skill of Silla architects and the depth of the Buddhist faith.

than the inhalation, we begin counting, assigning a single number to each breathe cycle. Count only to ten and then resume at one. Practice this first for a period of five minutes daily in the morning and evening if possible. Add an additional five minutes each week until your sessions reach thirty minutes in length. Focus on your breathing, allowing all stray thoughts to vanish from your mind. After much practice, counting will become unnecessary and a state of total relaxation will be achieved.

Aside from the mental ramifications, the physical body also stands to benefit from the dedicated practice of meditation. By lowering the body's metabolic, heart and respiratory rate, a physiological state of deep relaxation is induced. In addition, anxiety and tension have been linked to the blood's lactate level. It has been found that this chemical concentration is substantially reduced, as much as four times, in the person meditating. The skin's resistance to mild electrical currents, decreasing during times of emotional stress, increases as much

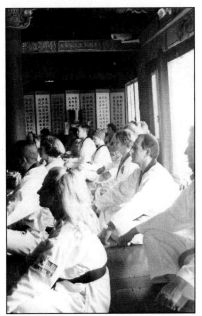

A group of students from the United States Taekwondo Association under the direction of Grand Master Richard Chun, sitting Zen meditation at the Pulguksa temple in Korea.

as four hundred percent during reflective practice. These are but a few of the physical manifestations of meditation and still there is much to be discovered.

Lastly, as we have seen, meditation can be used as a spark to ignite the fires of ki that burn within all living things. While in Korea, some fellow martial artists and I had the privilege of studying *Tjan Tjin Ho Hup* with a group of Buddhist priests. This advanced form of meditation is meant to heat one's internal ki furnace, ultimately leaving the practitioner less susceptible to illness and disease. We had been heading north, traveling along the coast all day and well into the evening, when we arrived at a small seaside village. Korea was experiencing their annual monsoon season and the night was incredibly hot and humid. Our travels with Masters Jong Chul Lee, Won Mo Jang, and Yoon Jai Cho had already proven to be a truly enlightening experience and we eagerly anticipated the promise of the following day. Next morning, before dawn, we were awakened by the crash of the surf pounding on the beach. The weather that morning was surprisingly clear and cool and the smell of salt air invigorating. We were a few miles from the thirty-eighth parallel—the imaginary boundary line separating North and South Korea. I lay awake, our small room separated from the outside by a pair of rice-paper doors, taking in the morning sounds of the awakening village. Shortly after donning my dobok, I joined the others who were stretching out on the beach in preparation for our workout. Once we were all assembled, the masters led us, double file, through the village's narrow streets, eliciting wide-eyed stares from the local citizens. Our destination was an ornate Buddhist temple perched among the rocks of the rugged sea wall. We climbed the steep, stone stairway carved from the bedrock in the side of the hill leading to the entrance that stood open facing the East Sea. Once inside, we formed two rows facing what we supposed was an altar of sorts, aflame with dozens of candles and statues of Buddha. Master Jang, speaking as he typically did through an interpreter, commanded us to assume a horse stance.

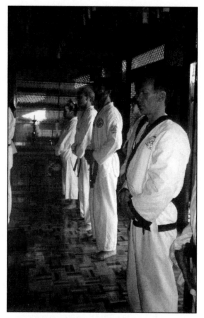

Practicing Tjan Tjin Ho Hup at a Buddhist temple near the 38th parallel in Korea.

We were then instructed to place our hands on our thighs, palms facing up forming a circle with our thumbs and index fingers. Through partially closed eyes, we began our structured breathing; inhaling for five seconds, pushing the air down into our tjan tjin, holding it for five seconds and then exhaling for a slightly longer period of time. Tjan Tjin Ho Hup and the mental concentration it required was evidenced by the perspiration dripping from our faces. Time evaporated as I allowed stray thoughts to flow in and quickly out of my consciousness in an attempt to achieve a state of no-mind. I began to feel my abdominal region grow warm, urging an unrestricted flow of ki to surge through all the major meridians, eventually terminating in my extremities. Following our meditation, a state of heightened awareness permeated the moment as we sat cross-legged, hands clinched tight over our knees, drinking in the words of a Buddhist minister as she spoke to us of Zen philosophy and how it related to life and the martial arts.

Understandably, it is no simple matter remaining immune to the mystical and suggestive powers of meditation while training deep within the land of taekwondo's origin. From the mountain retreats of the Hwarang to the ornate monasteries standing in mute testimony to a continent's profound belief in Zen Buddhism, hints of the connection between meditation, Asian history, and the martial arts abound. Consequently, with millions of the global population practicing this reflective art, is it any wonder that it would eventually gain acceptance in the West? Meditation offers the layperson a platform for enlightenment through self-realization if only for a short time. On the other hand, while the martial artist finds meditation a necessary tool in amplifying technique and mental acuity, the beneficial effects it bestows on mind and body extends into every minute of waking life. Presenting a relaxed and controlled demeanor in stressful situations allows the practitioner to be relied upon to lead and arrive at logical decisions. Having the ability to react quickly and without restraint can often mean the difference between success and failure in daily life. Moreover, by drawing on Eastern philosophies founded in the distant past and using them as templates for every day living, we can expect positive results in almost anything we set out to accomplish. Meditation, therefore, if practiced diligently in conjunction with contemplation, visualization, and rejuvenation of the vital life force, can set the stage for achievements built on mindful intent and spiritual self-fulfillment.

CHAPTER 12

Personal Defense: Shields and Weapons

"Just one more present and I'm done," thought Terry as she made her way to an escalator. Christmas shopping at the Miracle Mall was always an exhausting experience with the crowds of people and the long checkout lines. A gift for the kids almost fell from her arms as she made a quick turn into the video store. She would buy her husband that martial arts movie he had always wanted to complete his collection of Bruce Lee films. She paid the clerk and made her way past the nativity ornaments to the big, sliding glass doors at the mall entrance. Stepping outside, Terry noticed that a light snow was falling, dusting the waiting cars of the holiday shoppers. As she stepped from the curb, she caught a brief glimpse of a group of women standing in a pool of light generated by one of the overhead flood lamps. Not twenty feet in front, shopping bags hanging from each arm, shuffled an elderly lady leaving a trail of footsteps in the deepening snow. Out of the corner of her eye, she caught a series of abrupt movements as two shadows dashed from between a row of parked cars straight for the older woman. Against the backdrop of the enormous parking lot, the women's feeble screams were lost in the cold night air as first one man and then the other grabbed at her parcels. Everything seemed to be happening in slow motion. Terry froze in her tracks watching as the men, seizing a further opportunity, began running towards her.

Nothing seemed easy in the rough and tumble world of business these days. Lee and his team assumed they had been doing a good job on the expansion project; the client was happy, they were on schedule and there were no cost overruns...until this morning when he arrived at work to find a message on his desk from one of the company's vice presidents requesting a conference. "No good could come of a meeting with this self-proclaimed captain of industry," he thought candidly. Mr. Hindes had a reputation throughout the division for being a rude and arrogant man. He was known for cutting conversations off in mid sentence and discouraging any sort of initiative. Lee hesitated as he punched in the extension number on his telephone. "Half a day, Reston?" said the gruff voice at the end of the line. It was him and already he was starting—not a good sign. Looking at his watch, Lee registered that it was 7:23 A.M. "You wanted to see me, sir?" "Yes!" rasped Hindes, undoubtedly masked in a fog of cigarette smoke. "It's about that new idiot you have working for you...what's his name? Oh yeah, Davidson. Where did he get his engineering degree from, some toy factory?" "He graduated from M.I.T., top of his class, Mr. Hindes. He's really quite good considering that he's..." "I don't care where he came from," spat the VP, his temper flaring. "All I care about is where he's gonna go if he doesn't shape up. Can't you do anything right?" Hindes, knowing full well that Lee had hired the young honor student, continued his tirade. He alluded to Davidson's proclivity for working late, thus making him look bad when he left early to play golf. "Get down here right now! We need to take care of this thing immediately. I have a big game today!" Lee could feel himself turning red, his blood pressure shooting sky high. He was experiencing feelings clear across the emotional spectrum from intimidation to anger. Reluctantly, he rose from his chair. Taking the doorknob in his hand, he began to mentally prepare himself for what lay ahead.

Katy couldn't imagine what was taking her mother so long. She was usually waiting right there by the mailbox at the entrance everyday when school let out. Now it was almost four o'clock and still no mom. She could hear the staccato sounds of someone sweeping the long hallway behind her as she peered through the glass door hoping to see some sign of movement. "Everything okay, honey?" She looked up into the jolly face of Mr. Huston, the school custodian, as he emptied his dustpan preparing to leave for the day. "Yes, everything's fine. I'm just waiting for my mother to get here." "Well, stay inside the lobby until she does," he exhorted. Katy promised she would but after another fifteen minutes she began to grow concerned. "What if she's sick and can't leave the house?" she worried. Making a decision, she pushed opened the door and ran down the short flight of granite steps, through the wrought iron gate and out onto the sidewalk. Being nine years old wasn't easy sometimes, especially in a new neighborhood. Katy turned first one way and then the next. She began walking apprehensively in what she thought was the right direction to her home. At first, Katy didn't notice the yellow sedan as it slowed and then lazily matched the cadence of her youthful pace. The car sped up a little and pulled over to the curb a few car lengths ahead. The driver's side door opened and a woman wearing sunglasses with her hair pulled back got out. Looking pensively around, she knelt down as the little girl came adjacent to her and stammered, "You, ah, lost sweetheart?" No answer. "I said are you lost?" Still no answer. Katy clearly remembered her parents telling her never to talk to strangers. "Hey, look at me. Your mother sent me to get you!" said the woman. Katy was galvanized. What if mom had sent her? "Do you know where my mother is?" asked the little girl, finally breaking down. The woman looked relieved. "Sure I do. Hop in. I'll take you to her right now!" Slowly, she put out her hand to take Katy's.

Truth be told, all of us, man, woman and child alike, hope never to find ourselves in a scenario even remotely similar to those portrayed above. Unfortunately, in a world sometimes based on greed, perceived power and self-interest, occurrences of this nature too often exist. How an individual defends himself in situations similar to these is a function of many things. Factors such as physical ability, mental acuity, and maturity all come into play. It is not enough merely to be strong and full of youth only to lack the essential strategic skills required to reverse a potentially disastrous happening. Nor is it sufficient to possess remarkable intelligence only to fall short of the strength necessary to quell an opponent. Defining, choosing, and developing strategies needed to address the challenges we must face in daily life, of whatever magnitude, is the essential difference between the doctrines of self-defense and personal defense.

Unlike self-defense, where one is generally expected to rely on a limited series of physically choreographed maneuvers in the hope of overwhelming an adversary, personal defense is all encompassing. Being aware of the surrounding environment, setting the mind, breathing correctly coupled with ki projection, knowing where and when to strike and with how much force, then finally mounting an appropriate assault are all tools for personal defense. As any skilled tradesman can attest to, it is essential that one match the proper tool to a specific job in order to achieve acceptable results. Clearly, an experienced carpenter would not use a hammer to drive in a screw just as he would not rely on a saw to pound in a nail. Likewise, the martial artist must become aware of the correct technique to use in a certain defensive situation if his training is to be effective. It stands to reason that taekwondo, by virtue of its traditional code of honor, uncompromising physical training, and holistic philosophy concerning mind, body, and spirit, stands apart from other disciplines. In his book, *Promise and Fulfillment In the Art of Taekwondo*, Sang Kyu Shim states, "the taekwondo program inculcates the accompanying mental set that precludes inhuman or unlawful exercise of acquired physical power, but also invests the highest standard of social and personal mores guiding the proper use of power." In short, taekwondo contains the necessary shields and weapons required to protect against almost any situation presented in daily life.

The ancient Hwarang ethical code clearly emphasizes the use of good judgment where the taking of life is concerned. Granted, when a person of lesser stature is threatened in a dark alley, little thought is given to the moral, ethical and legal issues raised by such an exigency. Still, in today's society there are laws the martial artist must abide by governing the acceptable level of force used in defending against a life-threatening attacker. Because most cultures recognize an individual's right to protect themselves, the use of reasonable force is largely legally acceptable, although common sense must prevail at all times. Therefore, it is safe to say that a defender may use whatever means necessary in defeating an armed assailant bent on inflicting serious bodily harm. On the other hand, if an innocent scuffle were to break out between two friends, one being a black belt, excessive force of this sort would, in all likelihood, be deemed ethically and legally unacceptable. In fact, it may result in criminal charges being brought against the martial artist.

Additionally, it is important to note that once an opponent has been disabled, the attack must cease with the injured party either being tended to or left in the hands of the proper authorities. Defending the weak or those unable to protect themselves is yet another eventuality the taekwondoist must be prepared for. In this case, the individual's right of self-defense is transferred to the protector in the eyes of the law. A plausible example would be coming to the aid of a senior citizen or a child who is clearly being threatened.

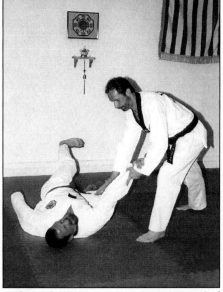

Concurrent with the traditional belts a martial artist earns over the course of his training, comes the added responsibility of acting with restraint and forethought. Therefore, before any defensive measure can be executed or level of force considered, a decisive plan of action must be decided upon. The choices available to us are detailed in the guidelines set forth by the Four Modes of Engagement. These stratagems, which escalate in complexity, offer the modern day warrior a combination of

Taekwondo contains an extensive arsenal of effective self-defense techniques. It is essential, however, that the martial artist gauge the perceived level of threat and refrain from the use of excessive force.

offensive and defensive tactics drawn from taekwondo's arsenal of shields and weapons. The blocks, kicks and punches of both a physical and spiritual nature represent these shields and weapons.

The first course of action consists of a strategy whereby we turn a deaf ear to threats, avoiding altogether those who would provoke an altercation. Refusing to be drawn into a confrontation is not the way of cowardice, but of maturity and self-control. Holding combat skills in abeyance based on a show of mercy is a sign of a true martial artist's confidence and humility.

The practitioner who chooses to cross the street rather than become entangled in a battle with a group of ruffians best exemplifies this mode.

Revolving around the use of wits and words, the second mode of engagement finds the practitioner attempting to negotiate a peaceful solution to a conflict by verbally sparring against an adversary. This technique combines both offensive and defensive skills since at times a conciliatory tone must be taken while at other times it may become necessary to appear irrational, even going so far as to feign sickness. Women, in particular, can use this tactic to great advantage. A warning of the possible consequences from a queasy stomach or the likely transmission of a life-threatening disease can cause a potential assailant to retreat rather quickly! Again, the ultimate goal is the avoidance of physical violence by defusing a dangerous situation through discussion before it is given an opportunity to spiral out of control.

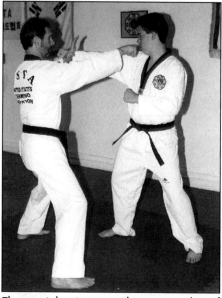

The martial artist must cultivate a number of strategic defensive skills in addition to those of a physical nature.

The third mode of engagement assumes the practitioner has lost the opportunity to resolve a threat by flight or negotiation and may, quite literally, be backed into a corner with no chance of escape. Furthermore, it is determined that the attack was not premeditated and that the assailant is unarmed and not likely to offer resistance once subdued. Following this quick but thoughtful analysis of the situation, a decision is made that a confrontation is imminent and that a measured physical response is clearly warranted. Reaching into the defensive toolbox of the martial artist, the practitioner may decide upon an appropriate countermeasure such as a nonlethal wrist lock or submission hold. These techniques are intended to disable an attacker with little or no prolonged effect on their well being, but must be maintained until assistance arrives or the proper authorities take control of the situation. While total commitment to the technique in question is essential, the goal is one of submission rather than defensive safety at any cost. Being accosted by someone under the influence of alcohol may qualify as an example of this scenario.

The Korean philosophy Il Kyuk Pil Sul or "first strike, swift and complete," sets the tone for the final, and admittedly, most severe mode of engagement. This tactic must be approached with the utmost seriousness and pursued only after all other attempts at pacification have failed. Its centerpiece is the irrevocable commitment to an opponent's total destruction in combat, further augmented by the defender's acceptance that he too may very well suffer injury in the process. While this technique may at first appear disturbing to the Western mind, it is this very demonstration of indomitable spirit that compelled the Hwarang and samurai warriors of the past to enter into battle with such ferocious resolve while seeming to harbor little or no concern for their own safety. Uehara Seikichi, headmaster of the Okinawan style of *Motobu-Ryu Udun-Di,* puts this strategy into perspective through this colorful statement: "When you fight an opponent, be ready to fill two graves, yours and your opponents." The Japanese also have a phrase describing this mind set as noted by Dave Lowry in his column, The Karate Way. *"Ikken hisatsu* is not a testosterone-fueled kamikaze charge. It is not a matter of bravado or phony patriotism or machismo. It's a calculated, logical and premeditated attack. It means accepting coldly and with knowledge aforethought that someone will die in the next few moments. It means that you are willing to attack with total commitment." He continues, "Ikken hisatsu is the realm where life and death come together." Clearly, through this statement, the Four Modes of Engagement are not unique to taekwondo, but embraced globally by the majority of traditional martial disciplines.

Should it become necessary to apply this final mode of engagement in a combat situation, it is essential that we take into consideration another issue surrounding its successful execution.

Assuming the martial artist will be given only one opportunity to deliver a single, devastating technique, all the knowledge learned in the martial tradition must crystallize and be poured into the moment. Otherwise, any plan of action will become nothing more than an empty threat—a powderless round.

Awareness. How many times have we noticed people walking the street, eyes downcast, buried deep in thought? It is important to know what is happening around you—who is present, what the terrain is like, and if there is room to maneuver if necessary. If you feel threatened, slowly turn your head side to side as you walk, scanning the periphery. Being aware does not mean you are paranoid. It simply makes you cognizant of your environment.

Environment. Should a confrontation ensue, use the environment to your advantage. Remain on high ground. Keep the sun to your back. Do not permit yourself to be backed into a corner but also do not allow an attacker to take up a position behind you. Seek illuminated areas if it is to your advantage. Use whatever implements are available as weapons (trashcan lids, tree branches, etc.) Conversely, recognition of your environment in everyday living can perhaps lead to the discovery of areas, at work, school or home where you may feel a more productive sense of creativity or restfulness.

Focus. The importance of focus to personal defense in a combat situation cannot be over-emphasized. If, in truth, we must destroy our opponent with a single blow, then that blow must be well placed and accompanied by all the ki energy, speed, and strength the body can muster. Furthermore, we cannot allow the surroundings or circumstances to impede our concentration on the selected point of impact.

Presence of Mind. This is the ability to remain calm in the face of possible disaster. Probably one of the most difficult psychological attributes to display, presence of mind can mean the difference between panic and the ability to execute a defensive technique appropriate to the situation. Succumbing to panic can result in defeat when staring into the eyes of an attacker. All the lessons we have acquired in the safe confines of the dojang can dissipate in the heat of the moment. It is therefore essential to cultivate the ability to remain calm and focused in battle as in life. This can be accomplished through meditation and diligent practice.

Correct Breathing. Proper breathing sets the rhythm for any orchestrated plan of attack. The exhalation of breath must accompany all hand or foot techniques if they are to be effective. Deep breathing will refuel the body, permitting it to endure extended periods of physical motion without exhaustion. On the other hand, utilizing correct breathing techniques during life's stressful moments can have a profoundly soothing effect both mentally and physiologically.

Use of Ki. Different schools of thought attach varying degrees of importance to the worthiness of ki energy during combat. Some argue that it is virtually impossible to affect an opponent in any way using the vital life force, going so far as to declare it black magic. Others claim to possess the power to repel an attacker without so much as laying a hand on their adversary. Most martial arts, however, tend to encourage some form of ki development in their training. Traditional taekwondo, hapkido, and aikido in particular, subscribe heavily to the existence of ki and its cultivation. As a holistically oriented aspect of personal defense, ki energy can be used as a tool to intimidate an opponent through the use of the kihop. Internal ki energy, channeled to and through the martial artist's weapon of choice, be it hand or foot, staff or sword, can multiply its effectiveness many fold.

Thus far, our discussion concerning personal defense has primarily centered on strategies targeted at countering the human predator. But what of the hidden threats posed by forces that come disguised in the form of the food we eat, the air we breathe and the negative thoughts projected by others. These threats can prove equally harmful to the body as a physical assault. Since the ultimate goal of any defensive measure is to protect the individual, how then does the doctrine of personal defense relate to these other harmful forces?

In a practical sense, short of relocating to a more wholesome climate, there is little one can do about the pollution of the air so prevalent in today's urban centers. Becoming an advocate for environmental protection can, in some small way, assuage the naturalist in all of us. However, it is largely the responsibility of the individual to shoulder the burden of conserving the earth's resources and use them wisely. Once again, this is a reflection of the holistic attitude the modern day warrior must learn to cultivate to benefit himself and the community at large. The body is a vehicle that is driven by the engine of the mind and being so, must be finely tuned and fed the proper fuel. Therefore, removing from our diet foods and beverages that are unnatural or simply unfit for consumption is yet another aspect of personal defense. It is not difficult to identify foodstuffs that offer little or no nutritional value. Chemicals such as nicotine and alcohol should be eliminated altogether if the practitioner takes their martial arts training seriously. Subsequently, accepting nutritional responsibility and tailoring it to the lifestyle pursued by the martial artist is yet another shield in the arsenal of personal defense.

While invisible to the eye, assaults to the spirit can prove even more damaging than those to the body. While scars of a physical nature will heal with time, a crushed spirit may never revive. For this reason, it is imperative to defend against the negative thoughts and actions of those who would discourage independent thought. Maintaining a positive attitude in the face of negative criticism is difficult at best and must emanate from within. It is important to keep in mind that the Taoist belief in the duality of opposites (um and yang) can bolster the knowledge that joy and prosperity are certain to replace sorrow and failure. This outlook does not require the martial artist to passively accept his lot in life, thinking it static and unchangeable. Indeed, the opposite is true. Through the cultivation of ki, coupled with meditative visualization and positive actions, the practitioner can conquer life's trials and tribulations, appearing both confident and self-assured in the process. Developing these qualities is vital to the overall health and welfare of the individual's mind, body, and spirit.

Now that we have become more familiar with the resources available to the martial artist through the diligent and holistic study of personal defense, let us reexamine the scenarios put forth at the beginning of this chapter to see what methods our three defenders have chosen to use in their battle for psychological and physical survival.

Terry, while not a martial artist herself, was given some abbreviated lessons by her husband, a black belt instructor in taekwondo. After twenty-five years of being surrounded by the martial arts, she could not help but pick up a few techniques here and there. He had demonstrated a tactic whereby a simple car key, with its shaft protruding through the space between the index and middle fingers, can act as an extremely effective weapon once a fist is made. Knowing it was late and she was alone, Terry took her keys from her bag after paying for the video, following the drill she had practiced so many times before. Once outside in the parking lot, she instantly became aware of her environment noticing the weather, illuminated areas and her proximity to other people at all times. Because she was scanning the space in front of her, she was quick to sense an emergency in the making. Surprising even herself, Terry maintained her presence of mind as the two men advanced on her. Frightened, she took a few deep breaths, realizing there was no way to avoid a confrontation. Seconds passed and a firm commitment was made in her mind to self-preservation. As the first assailant came within reach, Terry drew back the hand holding the key, swinging it in a great arc and ripping the man's face as metal came in contact with flesh. Clutching the wound, he went down on his knees. Turning, she quickly and deliberately delivered a devastating front kick to the second opponent's groin, causing him to fold up in pain as well. By this time, the entire area was alerted and people came running towards her from all directions. Calmly returning the elderly woman's belongings to her, Terry picked up her own parcels and proceeded to her vehicle. Glancing in her rear view mirror as she pulled out of the parking space, she made note of a large group of women pummeling the fallen thugs as mall security began to arrive in force.

Lee, on the other hand, was a practicing taekwondoist who not only held numerous championships pursuant to the sport side of the Korean discipline, but was well versed in the spiritual aspects of the martial art as well. Wanting to use the environment to his advantage, he had requested that Mr. Hindes meet with him in the cafeteria over a cup of coffee. This effectively removed his opponent from the comfortable surroundings of his own office, placing them both on neutral ground. From his years of sparring in competition, he had learned the importance of correct breathing in stressful situations. And so, as he walked down the hall towards the elevator, he began a series of breathing exercises aimed at calming the mind and strengthening his internal ki. Hindes became somewhat ill at ease as he noticed the fierce look in the eyes of this young man sitting across the way from him. Maintaining presence of mind and not allowing himself to lose his temper in any way, Lee dominated the conversation. While remaining respectful and humble, he laid out his concerns in a logical and firm manner while defusing the vice president's heated retorts at every turn. Lee realized that this discussion would not permanently alter Mr. Hindes' demeanor. But in winning the verbal sparring match, he left the table confident in the fact that he had done the honorable thing in sup-

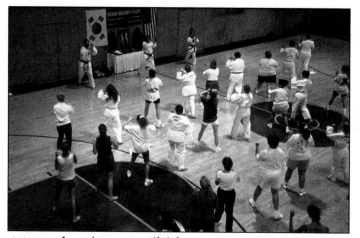

Women often take part in self-defense courses with the hope of not becoming a victim to senseless violence.

porting Davidson even though he had done nothing wrong to begin with. Mr. Hindes did concede that maybe he had been a little hasty in his judgment of the new employee and left, chain smoking, grumbling something about having to be "on the green" in short order.

By now, little Katy was totally confused and very frightened. Somewhere in the back of her mind she remembered the yellow belt she held in karate, but was too scared to recall any of the defensive techniques she had learned in class. At the present time, her reality consisted of her fear and this ominous woman in sunglasses kneeling before her. Still, somewhere in her consciousness, she heard the voice of her instructor as she urged her young students to scream as loudly as possible should they ever feel threatened by a stranger. Just as the woman's fingers touched Katy's wrist, she broke free of her stupor and began crying for help. Pulling free of the molester's grip, she turned and began to run down the sidewalk towards the busy main street. Sensing the hopelessness of the situation, the woman jumped back in her car, leaving the scene with a squeal of rubber and a cloud of dust. Not moments later, a license plate number was being jotted down by a startled pedestrian whom the speeding vehicle had narrowly missed hitting. Looking up from his note pad, Mr. Huston, the school custodian, noticed the terrified little girl who had been waiting for her mother minutes before, running directly towards him.

In the final analysis, personal defense can be viewed as a comprehensive and scientific approach to self-defense. Each element must be taken into account before any effective response can be mounted. Consequently, the required skills must be practiced in such a way so as to be carried out efficiently and without conscious thought. An ill-considered tactic will not only dilute the final result, but could spell disaster in the long run. Furthermore, it should come as no surprise to find a common holistic thread running through the entire doctrine of personal defense. This is a direct reflection on the art from which these fundamental strategies are drawn. The shields and weapons so abundant in taekwondo's arsenal are a manifestation of a nation's will to survive against insurmountable odds. Therefore, by diligently applying the techniques unique to this Korean martial art, the practitioner can feel secure knowing that they are well prepared for any situation that may be encountered in daily life.

CHAPTER 13

The Warrior Way

Over the course of global history, warfare has played a significant role in the rise and fall of civilizations. These shifts in the geopolitical fabric were often a result of irreconcilable conflicts, fueled by imperialistic desires, racial discontent, or religious dissension. Differences in ideology invariably escalated into violent action instigated by tribes, clans, or nations antagonistic towards one another. Even in these "enlightened" times we live in today, there is no shortage of rationalizations to explain away this aggressive behavior. Some claim that armed combat is the only real method for solving disparities among men. Others posit that mankind must mature well beyond this current stage of evolutionary adolescence before any alternative to war can be found. Still there are those who patiently await an act of God to remove this fatal flaw in the human condition. But rather than explore the tedious political ramifications and mechanics behind war itself, it is the motivations and qualities of the human instrument, traditionally used by kings and generals in their lust for victory, that we are concerned with here.

From the age of clubs and stones to the present day use of laser-guided tactical weapons, the warrior's mission on the battlefield has remained the same: to gain physical or ideological dominance over his opponent and survive. How this is accomplished is a function of the combatant's training, courage, and tenacity. But to say that survival lies exclusively in a formal military education coupled with nerves of steel would be inaccurate at best. For hidden in the heart of every true warrior is an ingredient that defies quantification. It is a quality that radiates from the center. It lives in the soul and represents the essence that drove the Hwarang, the samurai, the crusader, and the native American Indian to perform feats that will be retold for centuries. It is the warrior spirit. Is this advanced state of martial consciousness identifiable as an attribute common in all people?

Hardly! In order for a warrior to be recognized as such, there are certain fundamental parameters that must be met. He first must practice patience and courage, knowing when to hesitate and when to advance. He must show mercy as well as ruthlessness in battle. He must be willing to face death as readily as he would be to deliver it upon another. Above all, he must not stray from his mission, demonstrating the same ferocity and determination to see each task through to its logical end, no matter how distasteful or appealing. How has the warrior spirit been exemplified over time, and who can we turn to as a model? Furthermore, is it possible that these virtues are genetically embedded by dynastic rite, or can they be acquired over time through constant training? Questions such as these are sometimes best answered through example, either by manifestations of heroic distinction, or in an uncompromising series of noble principles. The former can be found written on the pages of history. However, through the window of experience, we can view the notable deeds of those who have truly exemplified the warrior spirit. Conversely, answers to the latter have been inscribed in a set of philosophies that, if followed in earnest, will lead us on the path to genuine virtue. Wu Wei, an author and scholar of Chinese I Ching philosophy, states that, "By studying the sayings that have survived the test of centuries, we gain wisdom. By learning the deeds of our ancient heroes, we gain inspiration. Wisdom, coupled with inspiration, leads to good fortune and supreme success." Through these words we can appreciate the inspirational value in tracing the footsteps of our ancestors of the martial arts tradition.

The life and times of the Asian warrior has, over the decades, become popularized in film and television. Images of samurai, wielding razor-edged katana, leap from the screen to the delight of action-hungry audiences resulting in big profits at the box office. While this is understandable, given the benign entertainment value of martial arts in the cinema, it should be remembered that classic fighters were mere men susceptible to moods and illnesses just like any other. Often these soldiers were forced to endure adversities in the line of duty far in excess of those faced by the average citizen. Hunger, disease, and extreme weather conditions all went into molding the character of the individual. Some were mercenaries, willing to divide their allegiances for monetary gain; others displayed fierce loyalty to king and country with no thought of self-aggrandizement. One such example was that set by Kwan-ch'ang, a Hwarang warrior, already an assistant general under his father, General P'umil, at age sixteen. Following a number of setbacks during an important battle with Paekche in 660 A.D., Kwan-ch'ang's father requested that he rally his forces and rouse the troops of the other generals. In the midst of battle, the boy warrior galloped into the enemy camp leaving a trail of vanquished adversaries in his wake. Kwan-ch'ang was taken captive and brought before General Kaebeck, commanding officer of the Paekche forces. Astonished by both the courage and youthfulness of the prisoner, the General exclaimed, "This is only a boy! Alas for us if we cannot match such courage. If these are the exploits of a boy, what must we expect from their men!" At this point, realizing the valor in the deed, the commander ordered the young man be allowed to return to his camp unharmed. But, no sooner had Kwan-ch'ang been released than he reentered the fray, spearing many opponents along the way. After being recaptured, as punishment, he was this time decapitated and his head sent back to the Sillian troops tied to his horse's saddle. Rather than being viewed as a tragedy, however, Kwan-ch'ang's father lifted the head from the saddle with the pronouncement, "My son's honor lives! I have no regret that he gave his life for his king." The Sillian army, deeply moved and inspired by such virtuous action, went on that day to obtain a decisive victory over the Paekche forces.

Yet an even more enduring example of the warrior spirit can be found some nine hundred years later in the accomplishments of Korean Admiral Yi Sun-sin, a man purported to be one of the world's greatest naval tacticians. Born in 1545, Admiral Yi is credited with the design and manufacture of the *kobukson,* the first armored battleship thought to be a precursor of the modern day submarine. Measuring 110 feet long and 28 feet wide, these early vessels came to be known as "turtle boats" due to a series of curved metal plates uniquely designed to protect the upper decks from attack. These plates bore a vague resemblance to a turtle. With firepower in the way of multiple three-inch cannon, the kobukson commanded the seas, able to interdict any ship afloat.

At the bow, arrows and smoke issued forth through an opening in the mouth of a carved turtle's head that doubled as a ram, adding to the warship's already intimidating appearance. Compared with its Japanese counterparts, the kobukson was considered to be one of the most highly developed battle plat-forms of its day. But more important to those living in sixteenth century Korea, was the role Admiral Yi Sun-sin played in the defeat of the invading Japanese forces over the turbulent years of 1592 through 1598. In 1590, with hopes of ending the treach-ery of rival warlords within his native society, Toyotomi Hideyoshi, the shogun of Japan, contrived to shift the attention of his detractors away from his administration with a planned attack on China. When Korea refused to participate in the scheme, Hideyoshi dispatched a force comprised of some three hundred thousand troops, lead by Generals Kato Kiyomasa and Konishi Yukinaga. Unprepared, both in personnel and weaponry, the country was overpowered by the opposing army causing King Son-Jo to flee into exile. Citing various diplomatic treaties with China, the Korean king enlisted the aid of Ming troops ultimately halting the momentum of the marauding invaders. Admiral Yi Sun-sin, through the judicious use of his small navy, wreaked havoc on the occupying troops by severing their supply lines causing the Japanese forces to retreat. In a determining sea battle that finally put an end to any hopes of a Japanese con-quest over China, Admiral Yi opposed a formidable force of one hundred thousand reinforcements in the waters off Korea's southern coast. Initially feigning retreat, his fleet turned, eventu-ally sinking seventy-one enemy vessels. As naval reinforcements joined in the melee, he aggressively continued his attack destroy-ing an additional forty-eight warships. Time and time again, through the use of a shrewd battle formation that came to be known as the "fishnet," the brilliant strategist repelled portions of the Japanese fleet that outnumbered his small Korean armada by a ratio of ten to one.

At times, Admiral Yi seemed almost prescient in his abilities to predict the enemy's maneuvers. On one occasion, after awak-ening from a dream in which he heard a robed man crying out, "The Japanese are coming!", he ordered his armada to quickly set sail. Before long, the warships encountered an enemy fleet and attacked with characteristic vigor, burning twelve vessels in the process. Through it all, Admiral Yi continued to display his typical courage by urging on the attack in spite of a bullet wound to his shoulder. Because of his patriotism, ingenuity in battle, and overt concern for the Korean naval forces, the commander became a highly decorated officer. But as the I Ching teaches us, decline must follow prosperity and for Admiral Yi Sun-sin, the tide was about to change.

Hideyoshi, realizing full well that any future assault on Korean territory would again result in defeat as long as Admiral Yi retained control of the waves, connived to strike at King Son-Jo's military hierarchy by planting a spy in its midst. And so it came to be that a Japanese soldier named Yosira, posing as a defector, slowly gained the confidence of General Kim Enug-Su by feeding him artificially useful bits of intelligence. When warned of an impending invasion by a sizable Japanese fleet, General Kim ordered Admiral Yi Sun-sin and his armada of turtle boats to set sail immediately and lie in wait for attackers. Yi, possibly sensing the deception, refused to follow the General's directive based on his knowledge of the hazardous terrain submerged beneath the expected point of engagement, waiting to rip the hull from any vessel that strayed in its direction. Once notified of the Admiral's decision by Kim, King Son-Jo wasted no time in his reply ordering that Yi Sun-sin be arrested and brought to Seoul in chains. Upon the recommendation of King's council, Won Kyun replaced Admiral Yi, despite all his courageous acts. He was beaten, tortured, and reduced in rank to a mere foot soldier. Even during these darkest of times, Yi did not complain, but rather continued to humbly execute the responsibilities of his new position. In 1597, with Admiral Yi safely removed from command, Hideyoshi seized the initiative, sending an invasion force of one hundred forty thousand men in hundreds of ships to once again ravage the war torn peninsula. Plotting the total destruction of the Korean Navy, the spy Yosira urged General Kim to dispatch Won Kyun and the meager fleet to meet the Japanese threat head on. Won Kyun, choosing to ignore the tried and true strategies of Admiral Yi Sun-sin, failed dismally in his attempt to defend his country. Panicking at the sight of a superior force,

Won Kyun retreated only to be captured and executed. Fearing for his nation's future, King Son-Jo wisely reinstated Yi Sun-sin to his former station. Exhibiting his customary loyalty and love for his homeland, the Admiral returned to command the twelve remaining ships without anger toward his former tormentors. Consequently, in what must have been a satisfying show of support, his former seamen rushed to his side as word spread of his new position. Once again, off the waters of Chin-Do Island, Admiral Yi reminded Hideyoshi of his awesome naval skills. Through tactics such as the "two salvo fire," the tiny Korean armada decimated a Japanese force that consisted of one hundred thirty three ships. The result was total retreat.

In 1598, after being harassed by members of the Korean volunteer army, cut off from provisions by Yi's vessels and disillusioned by the death of Hideyoshi, the Japanese troops were recalled home, but not before a final, ill-fated engagement. As the enemy was evacuating, Admiral Yi attacked, destroying nearly the entire remaining fleet. As he stood on the deck of his flagship, barking commands to his men, Yi was struck by a stray bullet. As years of military experience flowed away, mixing with his blood, Admiral Yi Sun-sin, in a final gesture of valor, was heard to say, "Do not let the rest know I am dead, for it will spoil the fight."

The examples set by Admiral Yi Sun-sin and the boy warrior, Kwan-ch'ang, while inspirational in a purely martial and historical sense, run concomitant with the lifestyles of those living in early Korea's highly volatile, pre-industrial society. But what of those of us today, secure and affluent by comparison, thriving in a world where wars are mostly fought by trained professionals in lands far removed from our daily routines? How will the cultivation of the warrior spirit, that valorous motive that separates the victor from the vanquished, the focused from the disillusioned, the impassioned from the cynic, benefit us? Even though the rattle of gunfire has come to define the chaos of conflict as we know it, there are wars, different from those fought with sword and spear, that the modern day warrior must face on a daily basis. Unlike their comrades in the trenches, these soldiers are difficult to discern since many and varied are their uniforms. They are the father working two jobs hoping to make ends meet, the single mother of four desperately attempting to feed a family, the businessperson financially wounded to the point of insolvency, and the teenager constantly weighing the pressures of popularity on the scales of sensibility. These determined warriors, bearing the burdens of today's realities, are no less courageous than those of the past and oftentimes must possess physical strength, mental acuity, and spiritual stamina far surpassing that of their ancient predecessors. However, it is not only those experiencing temporary misfortune that can benefit from following the warrior way. No, those with a predilection towards prosperity can further bolster their success through its precepts. For it is the nurturing of this warrior mindset, through the practice of taekwondo and its moral guidelines, that permits the sincere believer to enthusiastically endure life's battles in the face of seemingly insurmountable obstacles. To the modern day warrior, despair and surrender are unacceptable options.

What qualities then, are required for admittance into this elite cadre? Must an individual embrace violence as a prerequisite to warriorship? And, how does the diligent study of taekwondo aid in cultivating the warrior spirit? Taekwondo is a martial art that encourages and strives to instill courage, confidence, self-esteem and indomitable spirit in all its practitioners, regardless of age or gender. But rather than leave the masters and instructors of the art the chore of arbitrarily gathering philosophical doctrine to pass along to their students, the Korean martial art has given its leaders principles that stand in the long shadow of its classic heritage. These are the Five Tenets of Taekwondo.

The Five Tenets of Taekwondo

Courtesy

Integrity

Perseverance

Self-Control

Indomitable Spirit

Handed down through the ages, originating with the Hwarang and modified to meet our current social and moral standards, these tenets, while deceptively simple on the surface, are rich in virtue. By learning and embracing these noble principles, conjoined with a program of diligent, physical training, the martial artist is certain to capture the essence of the warrior way. One may wonder how attributes such as courtesy and integrity fit the mold of the raucous warrior slashing his way to victory. However, it is not the wars and weapons of past destruction that we are concerned with, but the act of adorning ourselves in a protective armor of virtue that can be called upon every waking minute of our daily life. Furthermore, embracing the violence of the sword would no more further our cause against emotional conflict than would turning our backs to the power of hope.

Even in light of their potential worth, it is surprising how many people, when asked, cannot accurately define the meaning of these five virtues. Let us then take each tenet singularly, determine its literal definition and assign it a precise value as a weapon in the arsenal of the taekwondoist turned modern day warrior.

Courtesy: A polite or considerate act or remark. Politeness of manners; especially politeness connected with kindness; civility.

Practical Application: Courtesy, when viewed through the eyes of the martial artist, begins with the bow of respect generously offered to seniors, fellow students and when entering and leaving the dojang. Most Westerners are not comfortable with this form of courtesy, finding it foreign and in some cases bruising to the ego. However, the taekwondoist, constantly aware of the potentially lethal nature of the art, learns early on to perform this simple demonstration of courtesy. A gratuitous, "Yes Sir" or "Yes Ma'am" almost always accompanies the bow. Over time, this verbal demonstration of respect is often carried outside the dojang with the student replying to strangers in similar fashion. Complimenting those who go out of their way to make us comfortable can also show courtesy. A parent taking a child to school, a spouse preparing a meal, or a pupil receiving an outstanding report card are all worthy candidates for an encouraging word. But more correctly, an act of courtesy should stem from nothing more than an innate desire to communicate thanks to another human being with no thought of reciprocity.

Integrity: The quality or state of being of sound moral principle; uprightness, honesty, sincerity.

Practical Application: Integrity is the "silent tenet" in that it needs to be practiced internally and is often invisible to others. It is the framework on which all the other tenets ride. In cultivating integrity, we have only one master to answer to—ourselves. Gauging our integrity index is easy. We must first ask: How do we act when we are alone or when no one is watching? If we find something of value on the street, do we make an effort to return it to its rightful owner, or do we keep it for our own? At work, do we apply ourselves fully to a given task, or do we hold back knowing our superiors are elsewhere at the time. In school, do we attempt a peek at our neighbor's work, thinking nobody will notice, or do we prepare on our own by studying in earnest? Integrity marks the difference between the individual who will take the morally correct path in questionable situations as opposed to the person who chooses the course of least resistance. One way the martial artist displays this principle is by practicing in private, away from the eyes of envious and congratulatory onlookers. Another is by training as hard as possible on the dojang floor since only the practitioner is aware of his own, ever-expanding limit. In short, at times it is both easy and tempting to fool ourselves. Integrity is an acquired safeguard that short circuits this human frailty and helps steer us through the maze of ethical behavior.

Perseverance: To continue on a given course in spite of difficulties and obstacles. To continue with a determination not to give up.

Practical Application: As important as it is to apply integrity in identifying our moral strengths and weaknesses, it is equally important not to become discouraged with our progress in the dojang as well as in daily life. The modern day warrior, in striving to live the warrior way, will eventually come to realize that there are many so-called friends, colleagues, and associates who may suddenly grow envious upon discovering another's attempt at living a superior life. This envy may manifest itself as negative criticism, feigned indifference, or mild hostility, causing the practitioner to become somewhat disenchanted about their training. At this point, the novice, as well as the experienced taekwondoist, may ask: Am I really capable of performing these techniques? Am I foolish to think that I can live up to the high standards required in the martial arts? Or, "My friend is right. I am too old for this and I don't have the time." It is then that the adherent must exhibit a true component of taekwondo: perseverance. One method of bolstering perseverance is by asking ourselves the correct analytical questions rather than those steeped in frustration. What effect has the practice of taekwondo had on the quality of my life? How do I feel today as opposed to a year ago? Has my attitude and the way I view life changed for the better? Answers to these queries often result in positive responses driving the practitioner even further along the rightful path—a path made easier by the maintenance of a strong body and soul. Consequently, it may behoove the practitioner to consider entering a program of physical exercise, such as weight lifting or jogging, as an adjunct to their formal training. Despite the obvious rewards intrinsic in such a program, demands placed on an already strained schedule are sure to further test one's ability to persevere. Life has a habit of throwing up detours on the road to a higher quality of life. However, persevering in the face of adversity, of whatever magnitude, is the sign of a truly dedicated martial artist.

Self-Control: Control exercised over oneself or one's own emotions, desires, or actions.

Practical Application: Imagine, if you will, a world whose inhabitants flagrantly act on primal instincts. Where raw emotion and unchecked desire run free. Where egotism displaces the common good. How long could such a civilization survive before falling victim to total anarchy? Fortunately for modern society, there is a defense mechanism built into the human psyche that minimizes the frequency of such unrestrained behavior. This moral dynamic, requiring both discipline and restraint as a foundation, narrowly defines the border between civility and chaos. Oddly, the most fragile of tenets is called self-control. Self-control is rather like the faucet on a bathtub—left tightly closed, the flow of water is totally restricted. However, if the same faucet is left open and forgotten, the water will fill the tub until it overflows, causing damage to the surrounding area. A haphazard effusion of emotion is similar in many ways. A stoic person can, at times, appear cold and apathetic, displaying little or no emotion, while on the other end of the spectrum, unfettered sentiment may be viewed as the rantings of a lunatic. Convention dictates that emotion and action are best expressed when they are contained within a socially acceptable envelope of behavior, the limits of which are set by self-control. This tenet, therefore, moderates an otherwise erratic current of conduct and is tempered by both maturity and wisdom. In the dojang, self-control can be observed most prominently during sparring practice. It is easy to attack an opponent with uncontrolled vigor, but asked to display good self-control coupled with appropriate technique as a portion of their training, the lower belt is often left bewildered. This is obviously done to avoid injury, but more importantly, to demonstrate one's ability to exhibit focus and restraint. Stopping a kick or punch just shy of the target is possibly the greatest manifestation of physical self-control in the martial arts. By the same token, in daily life, we practice self-control on a continual basis. Keeping our tempers in check when sitting in rush-hour traffic, maintaining presence of mind in a threatening situation, not becoming angry or upset when things do not turn out quite the way we had expected, are all worthy examples of self-control.

Indomitable Spirit: Last but certainly not least, indomitable spirit exists as the cornerstone of the proceeding four virtues and is best described by Larry W. Voorhees in an article published by the *United States Taekwondo Union Journal* titled, "The Five Tenets." In it he states, "Indomitable spirit is one's ability to stand up for what is right, no matter what the situation, no matter how great the cost, no matter how many or how powerful the adversaries...and being certain that you will prevail." Furthermore, since this final tenet continues to play such a major role in Korean culture, and thus the national martial art of taekwondo, the following chapter has been dedicated to a full discussion of its merits. Suffice it to say that a martial artist lacking indomitable spirit can be compared to a swift blade without its edge.

By now it should be evident that the cultivation and perpetuation of the warrior way is not a recent addition to the civilized world, nor should it be construed as a passing fad or fancy. In truth, it is and has been a necessary factor in mankind's propensity for survival. In ancient times the list of enemies included wild animals, feuding families and finally, warring countries. While these physical adversaries continue to exist, their ranks have been expanded to include others. Becoming victimized by the pathogens of materialism, decadence, and greed has become a simple matter of complacency. Moreover, these malignant qualities must be respected as the formidable weapons they are. They are just as devastating as the swords and flaming brands wielded by Hideyoshi and General Kaebeck. Often, we innocently forgive these actions by our peers based on the mistaken belief that this behavior is not only inevitable, but acceptable in limited doses. However, by acknowledging and cultivating the warrior spirit through the diligent practice of the traditional martial arts, by heeding the accumulated wisdom of our ancestors, and by embracing the five tenets of taekwondo, hope begins to unfold before our very eyes. This view can frequently be obstructed by trepidation, laziness, or despair and may require a complete philosophical reversal to overcome. Subsequently, by recalling the integrity, perseverance, and indomitable spirit exhibited by these courageous warriors, we begin to perceive that the light just over the horizon is not merely the glow of knowledge, but the silhouettes of warriors who have come before.

CHAPTER 14

Indomitable Spirit: The Power to Prevail

Perhaps the most visible example of indomitable spirit in recent martial arts history can be attributed to the late Bruce Lee. Aside from a wildly successful career as a film star and Hollywood television actor, there is little doubt that this legendary figure will be memorialized as one of the greatest martial artists of our time. At age thirteen, initially seeking a means of self-defense, Lee began the study of *wing chun,* a form of Chinese gongfu, in his native Hong Kong under the tutelage of the famous master, Yip Man. An ever-expanding passion for the discipline eventually lead to the founding of his own unique style of martial art that came to be known as *jeet kune do* or "the way of the intercepting fist." Having collected thousands of books on the subject and armed with a degree in philosophy, Lee was better suited than most in the martial arts community to assume a task that would befall him during one of the darkest periods of his life. In 1970, the young practitioner suffered a severe back injury causing his doctors to not only recommend that he remain in bed for months on end, but that he divorce himself from his beloved martial arts entirely. Where others would have easily acquiesced, Lee instead chose the path of the modern day warrior, clearly demonstrating what unmistakably came to be viewed as the ultimate statement of indomitable spirit. Sentenced to lay immobile, flat on his back for an interim of six months, Lee, with the help of his devoted wife, Linda, began transcribing his thoughts and techniques to paper. These notes, along with a number of rare philosophical insights and anatomical renderings sketched by the author himself, evolved into the *Tao of Jeet Kune Do,* a best-selling volume found in the library of every well-informed martial artist and considered to be the definitive document on the art developed by Lee. Following his recuperation, Lee once again turned his focus to furthering the art of jeet kune do, and in the process influenced the lives of thousands of future martial artists prior to his untimely death in 1973.

Practicing indomitable spirit on an individual level, as did Bruce Lee, is essential to the moral well being of any serious martial artist. Instilling this quality in the collective consciousness of a nation, however, is clearly another matter. But, that is exactly what a dedicated group of Korean masters did in the days during and following the wars of the twentieth century that decimated their country. Accordingly, in 1910, with the crystallization of the Japanese occupation came an era of repression and hardship all too familiar in the annals of Korean history. Until the splintered nation's liberation in 1945, the colonial government attempted to extinguish all vestiges of Korean culture. A distraught citizenry witnessed the burning of books, the rewriting of history, and the torture of jailed dissidents. Under Japanese rule, the practice of all native martial arts was strictly forbidden. Even though no formally organized instruction was available, various masters clandestinely continued transmitting the traditional forms to courageous students in an effort to breathe life into a dying national treasure. Consequently, taekwondo as we know it today, could have faced extinction if not for the indomitable spirit portrayed by a select group of veteran martial artists who endured harsh persecution under the reigning dynastic and imperialistic regimes. Taekkyon pioneer, Song Duk-ki, a student of master Im Ho who became legendary for "jumping over walls and running through the woods like a tiger," was one such martial artist who chose to train underground rather than surrender to the Japanese aggressors. Remaining in his homeland as an ardent supporter of the traditional martial arts, Song later admitted to a deep regret at the passing of his master before the final stages of his training was complete, feeling much of taekkyon had died along with him.

Another champion of the martial arts, Grand Master Won Kuk Lee, born on April 13, 1907 and the founder of Chung Do Kwan (School of the True Path) taekwondo, lends further credence to the rumors of this cruel treatment when he tells of the punishment inflicted on him and his family by the newly formed government shortly after independence. In an article published in *Taekwondo Times* he states, "I was arrested and accused by the government of being a leader of a group of assassins. My wife and family, my students Duk Seong Son, Yung Taek Chong and several others were beaten, tortured, and lynched by the government." These allegations surfaced only after Lee refused to embroil his five thousand students in the politics of President Syngman Rhee's Korean Republican party. Indeed, maintaining national pride and original technique when all society appeared to be crumbling around them took more than a modicum of indomitable spirit on the part of these brave martial artists. It was against the backdrop of these tragic events that the Korean martial arts secretly struggled to survive.

During this period even the Chinese were not immune to the political manipulations of a hostile government. Following the People's Revolution in 1949 and well into the 1960's, Chairman Mao Tse-tung saw the practice of gongfu as all that was evil in his nation. In an attempt to remove offensive philosophies and threatening techniques, the Communist leaders sanitized the martial art, transforming it instead into a modern theatrical form known today as wushu. As in Korea, there were those who remained steadfast to the art, practicing it behind closed doors. Through the perseverance of these faithful Chinese practitioners, the discipline of gongfu, with all its subsidiary styles, continues to evolve throughout the world as China's premiere martial art.

Before their unification under the banner of taekwondo, the native Korean martial arts, including taekkyon, kwonbop, and subahk, underwent a metamorphosis. Commensurate with the influx of foreign influences, these disciplines began to take on some of the nuances found in the open hand fighting art of Okinawan karate-do. This trend continued as exiled Korean masters traveling in neighboring China, or forced to work in Japan, returned to incorporate what they had learned into their own unique defensive styles. Founded in the early 1950's, the Korean art of *tang soo do,* referred to earlier as *hwa soo do,* became the beneficiary of just such an amalgamation. The depth of this alliance can clearly be seen in the Hangul/English translation of tang soo do that reads "the way of the China hand." In order to avoid interference from Japanese troops, originator

Hwang Kee relocated to Manchuria where, in 1936, he studied *guoshu*. Upon his return to Seoul, Kee established the Moo Duk Kwan, the "School of Martial Virtue," dojang in 1945, where he began teaching the discipline that would later become, by his own decree *Soo Bahk Do,* or "Way of the Striking Hand." Although it may not have been evident at the time, this contamination of classical form was not entirely negative considering the multiplicity of techniques in the contemporary Korean martial arts. In fact, as stated by Dakin Burdick in an article published in the *Journal of Asian Martial Arts,* Korean *kumdo, yudo,* and *yusul,* were patterned after their Japanese counterparts of kendo, judo, and jujutsu respectively. However, the real test of indomitable spirit came in 1946 when the masters of the six surviving kwans convened with the intent on creating a unified martial art and national sport with a distinctive Korean flavor.

Differing slightly in technical nuance and principle, this body consisted of the *Chung Do Kwan, Moo Duk Kwan, Yun Moo Kwan, Ji Do Kwan, Chang Moo Kwan,* and *Sang Moo Kwan.* Within a few short years, however, other schools would quickly surface. Although a number of attempts were made at reaching an agreement on a cohesive curriculum, it was not until 1955 that a successful strategy was reached on reviving the standards set by the Hwarang. Up to this period, the martial art we know today as taekwondo was in its elemental stage. Terms such as *Kong Soo Do* (Empty-Hand Way) and *Tae Soo Do* continued to dominate, bearing witness to the depth of foreign influence on the native, Korean martial arts. Consequently, to this day there remains some debate on the issue of who was actually responsible for coining the name of what is presently the world's most popular martial art and when. Some sources claim a simple phrase book was used in the selection of the three descriptive syllables. Although most now agree that it was General Choi Hong Hi, founder of the O Do Kwan dojang (School of My Way) in 1953 and the International Taekwondo Federation in 1966 who ultimately authored the term taekwondo, in 1955. General Choi is rightly credited with creating much of what we know today as traditional taekwondo and its unique set of hyung or forms originally known as the Chang Hon series. Moreover, Choi was responsible for staging the first kong soo do demonstration in the United States while training at Fort Riley, Kansas in 1949. Yet another contender claiming authorship of the name taekwondo, however, is Duk Seong Son, who came to inherit leadership of the Chung Do Kwan. Remaining at the forefront of the current public acceptance and Olympic recognition of "the foot, hand way," is Dr. Un Yong Kim, a man whose tireless efforts succeeded in catapulting taekwondo into the international arena. Under Dr. Kim's guidance, the World Taekwondo Federation with its headquarters at the Kukkiwon, has flourished and is currently recognized as the largest, global organization of its kind representing the art. Clearly, it can be said that the turbulent river of indomitable spirit continues to flow throughout the entire landscape of Korean martial arts history.

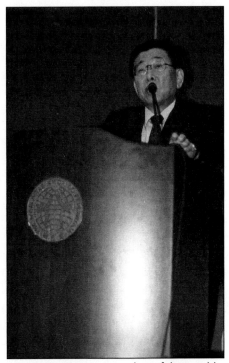

Dr. Un Yong Kim, president of the World Taekwondo Federation, is noted for his tireless efforts in forging taekwondo into an Olympic sport.

Having examined the available evidence then, a strong suggestion exists that if not for indomitable spirit, the surviving masters of post-war Korea may have decided against uniting the remaining kwans, thus effectively forestalling taekwondo as we know it today. Understandably, the hardships imposed during a time of war are enough to discourage and defeat even the most spirited among us and yet, the art prevailed. For the most part, we are fortunate to be living in a time of largely democratic rule unlike most of our Asian counterparts fifty years ago. Communism as an alternative form of government seems to have failed as many countries take their first steps toward a freer society. As a people, we enjoy the freedom to practice the martial arts as we individually see fit. Because of this, the virtues of taekwondo have been presented to a great many potential students who might not have been exposed to the art in the first place. For many of these practitioners, indomitable spirit has become a lifeboat in a tumultuous sea of hardship—a safety net allowing them to face misfortune in a controlled and hopeful environment. Fortunately, one does not need to be a master of the martial arts or live under the shadow of a despotic regime in order to enjoy the benefits bestowed by the cultivation of this precious virtue. On the contrary, for as many millions of taekwondoists as there are today, there are at least an equal number of examples depicting the reliance on indomitable spirit, some so dramatic that their accounting would be difficult to fictionalize. One story that comes to mind strikes at the heart of even the most stoic among us.

We will call him J.R., an active young boy of five innocently playing in his backyard one summer afternoon when he was stung by a bee. With no prior history of susceptibility, the insect's toxin quickly circulated through the child's body, throwing him into convulsions. After routinely checking on her son, his terrified mother rushed the boy to the hospital. By the time they had arrived at the emergency room, J.R. had slipped into unconsciousness and the doctors thought they might lose him. For weeks, the child remained in a coma, his parents sitting by his bedside around the clock, quietly reading and singing to him. Slowly, the child began to revive only to discover that his bodily functions were severely hampered. With much physical therapy, J.R. once again began to walk, but possessed the motor skills of a child half his age. After searching far and wide for a secondary remedy to thwart his disability, J.R.'s parents were told about taekwondo and the physical and mental virtues of the art. Every day, young J.R. would be brought to class by his mother and father and every day more progress would be made. His instructors patiently worked with him on basic stances and poom-se in an effort to retrain his recalcitrant muscles. Finally, following months of diligent practice, J.R. was ready to test for his yellow belt. His parents held their breath as the boy's name was called. Slowly, J.R. struggled to rise and made his way to his place in line. Step by step, strike by strike he labored through the examination until, upon completion, there was not a dry eye or still heart in the room. J.R. had done it! Triumphing over a severe handicap, he had earned, beyond the shadow of a doubt, his yellow belt. But he did not stop there as others may have. With the spirit of taekwondo instilled in his young soul, he persevered in his training, going on to earn his black belt.

As we can see, indomitable spirit comes to the aid of all, regardless of age, provided we exercise our acquired ability to draw upon this remarkable attribute in times of sincere need. Here we mean acquired in the sense that if we do not acknowledge the presence of this golden virtue through our efforts at diligent training in the spiritual aspects of taekwondo, we may never possess the capacity to borrow from it in the first place. Metaphorically speaking, it is impossible to draw water from a well whose existence we do not recognize. Furthermore, there is no underestimating the role courage plays in fueling one's desire to openly welcome this tenet in. One particular *I Ching* scholar, Wu Wei, observes, "Anytime anything happens to you that seems unfortunate, even if it is hurtful or takes something precious from you, see it in the light of a beneficial occurrence. It may not be immediately apparent what the benefit is, but by treating the event as though it occurred for your benefit, you will preserve your good feelings, and by acting in accord with those good feelings you will, as a direct result of cause and effect, bring about a happy result." If this is so it is because we sometimes need to be prodded or shocked into action given the idle nature of the human condition. In order to achieve the summit, we must sometimes navigate the valley or, quite literally, as in J.R.'s case, we may need to take one step back in order to make two steps of progress. Never giving up or allowing ourselves to give into the fear of failure, the frustration of effort, or the anger and anxiety of defeat is a major ingredient of indomitable spirit.

At this point one may ask, is the realization of indomitable spirit a function of diligent training or is proficiency in the martial arts a result of indomitable spirit? The correct answer to this riddle lies in the recognition of a synergy that develops over the course of a student's martial arts training; a synergy that is expressed as a ratio between an ever expanding amount of physical strength and confidence, compared with the will to triumph at any cost. Enhanced physical ability and self-esteem typically elevate the spirit, resulting in a cycle that tends to feed on itself. Likewise, the greater the enthusiasm and drive, the harder the pupil will push to attain new technical heights. Looking back at our chapter on measurable goals, we are reminded of the correlation between the practitioner's spiritual growth and the symbolic color of the belt they wear. To the white, yellow, and orange belt, coming from nothing to something is a dramatic gain. With each new technique comes the thirst for more. These increases in ability are generally accompanied by the desire never to miss a class; an emotion shared by many novices to the martial arts. Indomitable spirit truly begins to reveal itself during the training peaks and plateaus experienced by the maturing martial artist—the green, blue and purple belts. While the techniques taught during

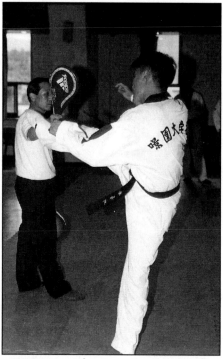

Korean martial artists train exceptionally hard to become proficient in taekwondo.

this period are charged with defensive value, they may appear somewhat lackluster considering that the wonder and innocence experienced by the lower belt is beginning to peel away. As the belt darkens, so should the taekwondoist's technical sophistication, physical prowess and spiritual density.

At red belt level, the techniques become even more complex with the introduction of advanced jumping and turning kicks. Even though these kicks may look simple when performed by an accomplished martial artist, they are, in fact, difficult to master and can prove daunting to the intermediate student. For many, especially the older pupil, this can be a discouraging time; a time when embarrassment and frustration may interrupt one's training. Enter indomitable spirit. For if the practitioner's mental and physical training programs have remained synchronous, the reservoir of resolve, largely untapped till now, can be counted on to supply the necessary hope to persevere. In order to remain consistent with this theory, however, modern day warriors must become acutely aware of their physical limits while always leaving room for improvement. Naturally, a compassionate instructor, sensitive to a student's goals and aspirations, will know when to push a trainee just beyond the edge of their current abilities. By the same token it would be unwise to expect a forty-year-old yellow belt to execute a sidekick (*yop chagi*) with the same trajectory and height as a teenager. In today's health conscious society, more and more mature men and women are embracing the martial

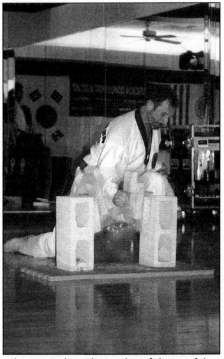

The internal resolve and confidence of the martial artist is tested with every breaking technique.

arts in the hopes of satisfying a longtime desire to become physically fit while developing defensive skills. It is therefore essential that the newcomer and veteran alike nurture patience and a sense of quality, not necessarily quantity, as fundamental prerequisites to a successful training regimen. What we mean by this is that special attention should be paid to mastering a given technique, first by dissecting and honing each individual component, followed by patient practice in a range of motion proportionate to the practitioner's physical abilities. Only after the kick or strike has been dynamically defined should an attempt be made at increasing both height and speed. If we set unrealistic standards for ourselves, it is likely that no amount of indomitable spirit will suffice in our efforts to succeed. Clearly, it is more desirable to perform fifty kicks with precision and deadly accuracy than one hundred of questionable form. By taking this qualitative approach to learning, the student will reap greater rewards in the long run.

Being on the dojang floor, where the fusion of mind and body actually takes place, offers further opportunities to call upon our internal resolve. *Kyuk pa,* or breaking, one of the more stunning examples of the power required in taekwondo is often a source of consternation among many students. However, accumulating inner strength and focus in the process, the surface of the object to be broken begins to take on a different character. It eventually diminishes in perceived physical mass and transforms, instead, into a spiritual boundary to be reckoned with. In more simplistic terms, this can be viewed as an act of mind over matter where fear must give way to unrestrained confidence. Why risk injury by breaking multiple boards or bricks with bare hands? For the very reason of sporadically testing one's indomitable spirit in a realistic domain. Approaching a hardened, concrete patio block, assuming a balanced stance, breathing in and focusing life-giving ki energy, then actually executing the break, allows the martial artist to demonstrate, not so much to others but to himself, the essential spiritual maturity demanded by taekwondo.

But what of injury? How does indomitable spirit help the student in this arena? Since taekwondo places such huge demands on the body's supportive tissue, the dedicated martial artist learns to live with the potential of injury on a daily basis. This situation is somewhat exacerbated by the fact that full contact sparring is encouraged and practiced in most forms of taekwondo. Even though the donning of protective equipment is mandatory under World Taekwondo Federation rules, the occasional strike can penetrate the best defense. Considering the very nature of the martial arts, getting hit becomes a fact of life. Consequently, assuming an injury entails nothing more than a pulled muscle or bruised finger, it is the habit of the majority of taekwondoists to view these as nothing more than minor inconveniences. However, an injury of marked severity should not be taken lightly and must be recognized for what it is. One should consult a physician and take every remedial action necessary in order to allay any recurring problems in the future. Histrionics or martyrdom where health issues are concerned clearly do not fall under the heading of indomitable spirit and can be considered foolhardy. Furthermore, once an immediate medical solution is administered, there are ways to turn an obvious disadvantage into a benefit. Along with twisted knees and sprained ankles come periods of recuperation where the student may temporarily be unable to train. Fortunately, certain injuries do not necessarily preclude the opportunity to participate on a different level. The medicinal effects of indomitable spirit are bountiful in that the pupil can attend class as an observer, stepping through the motions in their mind while viewing them first hand as performed by their fellow practitioners. In fact, simply being in the dojang surrounded by its sights, sounds, and smells can have a surprisingly restorative effect on the recuperating patient. But in the final analysis, it is the simple, sometimes unrelated issues that take their toll, chipping away at our resolve. Factors such as age, which has a bearing on flexibility, endurance and speed, and availability of time, dictated by work and family commitments, require substantial quantities of indomitable spirit to keep in perspective. By contrast, weight control and physically intensive concerns such as a disciplined exercise program can play equally into this equation. For instance, doing one hundred pushups as a prelude to training can drain the energy from even the most athletically gifted student, resulting in a feeling of unfounded incompetence. These demands must be viewed as the enemy within and tackled by indomitable spirit.

Warriors of all kinds throughout history, young and old alike, have relied on the fifth tenet of taekwondo as a tool in conquering life's adversities. A diversity of individuals ranging from mothers and sons to generals and film stars have found solace and victory in its pursuit. Indomitable spirit holds a sacred place in the classic Asian martial arts, but nowhere is its practice more evident than in the culture and social structure of Korea. Perhaps this is due, in part, to a history checkered by invasion and conquest. A proud people, the Koreans managed to persevere, rising from the ashes of war within a short span of

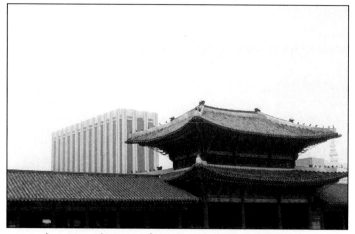

A modern Korea has risen from the ashes of war due, in no small part, to the tremendous resolve of its citizenry.

forty years into a modern economic power. Those not privy to the martial way might question what fervor could possibly have fueled the engine of Korean resolve so battered by time and oppression. An enlightened answer would be one that defines indomitable spirit not merely as the will to persevere at any cost in the face of insurmountable odds, but reveals a product consisting of many dynamics coming together simultaneously to create a greater whole. Included in this spiritual cloud are components such as courage, patience, honor, dignity and tenacity.

In its present form, the Korean martial art of taekwondo is not only a utilitarian defensive system, but a national symbol of the very spirit that supported the territorial unification of the three kingdoms in the seventh century. It spawned valiant military tacticians capable of brilliant strategic achievement and caused a splintered group of masters to join hands in a common goal of cooperation mirroring the values of their Sillian ancestors.

CHAPTER 15

Martial Art vs. Martial Sport

In the eyes of a gifted athlete there is perhaps no greater honor than to be standing in the spotlight as an Olympic gold medallist. Since 1894, when Pierre de Coubertin resurrected the games after an interruption of almost fifteen hundred years, it has been the dream of every competitor to achieve this highly regarded status. The Olympiad, first established in 776 B.C., has become the international forum for excellence in a variety of sports ranging from bobsledding and wrestling to figure skating and gymnastics. Now, after decades of effort on the part of a dedicated group of individuals, taekwondo has taken its place as a full medal Olympic sport alongside the Japanese discipline of judo. While many would assume this to be the greatest compliment a sport can be paid, the recognition of taekwondo by the International Olympic Committee as a competitive event has instead resulted in a great deal of debate between both traditional and modern factions of the art.

Critics contend that an emphasis on scoring points will eventually dilute the defensive value of taekwondo. Furthermore, it is claimed that taekwondo as a purely combative sport may discourage the adult population, a segment that may highly benefit from martial arts training, from participating. Seeing taekwondo in the Olympics may lead some adults to believe that it is difficult, if not impossible at an older age, to endure the bodily stress associated with full-contact competition. There is further concern that youngsters, too, may suffer from an overabundance of sport fighting by missing the spiritual and mental aspects so essential to the art of taekwondo. These issues, in addition to others we will examine, have led the serious martial artist to question just where sport ends and the art begins.

Supporters defending sport taekwondo note that the martial disciplines were not always reserved exclusively for defensive measures as many would assume. Rather, suggestions relating to the sportive aspects of the native Korean martial arts can be found in paintings on the walls of Muyong-chong, an ancient royal tomb located in a section of southern Manchuria once dominated by the kingdom of Koguryo. These murals, dating back to the first century, depict warriors sparring in stances oddly similar to those found in modern day taekwondo. Furthermore, there is proof that both taekkyon and subahk were viewed as recreational activities and as a means of physical fitness during the reign of King Uijong of the Koryo dynasty. The king, so impressed with the positive effect martial arts had on the body, used it as a yard stick in measuring the physical competency of his military commanders.

Later, as Confucianism pervaded the nation with its emphasis on state welfare through the nurturing of the superior man, the pugilistic aspect of the arts were swept into the background, remaining primarily as a form of entertainment at state festivals and government functions. A painting made by artist Hong Do Kim, a contemporary of the Yi dynasty, further supports this theory by showing two competitors engaged in free sparring for the apparent enjoyment of an audience congregated on the grounds of the royal temple. However, it was not until the sixteenth century, at a time when the Japanese were using the Korean peninsula as a stepping stone on their way to China, that the oppressed population again began to appreciate the brutal quality of their native martial arts. It was then that the military forces again relied on the fighting skills developed by bands of guerrillas and Buddhist monks who had secretly kept the martial arts alive in villages and monasteries throughout the land. Then, in the 1950's and 60's, as a nation desperately attempting to restore itself following the ravages of war, the Korean citizenry sought to highlight customs and traditions unique to their heritage. Thus, on the coattails of an inextinguishable desire to gain the respect of the industrialized world through the survival of their own country, came the creation of taekwondo as Korea's national sport.

It is important that we view this evolving phenomenon of taekwondo as a martial sport in the proper historical context so as not to confuse its true identity as the martial art that it is. Here was Korea, a country decimated by war, and hungry to revive its golden past. By taking what was already considered a natural resource and dressing it in the patina of nationalism, the Korean people solved a multitude of issues. First, it satisfied the need to develop a diversion, similar to Western football or boxing, that the population could enthusiastically rally behind. Secondly, the trim physical stature of the Korean people lent itself nicely to the flying kicks and other dramatic techniques associated with taekwondo, prominently marking them as the premiere practitioners of the sport. Even today, while many nations, including the United States, have made great inroads in their martial arts abilities, the Koreans continue to hold a distinct lead in this area.

This advantage bestowed pride on a people who, over the centuries, had been robbed of it and other privileges by foreign aggressors. This pride is enjoyed today in the form of accolades from the global athletic community who has come to recognize taekwondo as a truly Korean contribution to the diverse world of sports. Lastly, the unification of the various kwans or schools, following years of disagreement, may have been viewed by those involved as a microcosm of the events that eventually brought comparative stability to a nation wracked by internal and external conflicts.

Why then should an endeavor, apparently so worthwhile and wrought with historic precedence, come under fire at this time? In an effort to answer this question, one must understand that the above historical perspective is not intended to excuse or eliminate the need to reforge taekwondo. On the contrary, it is distinctly because of taekwondo's rapidly changing complexion, and partially due to its growing popularity as a diversionary pastime, that a careful re-evaluation of the art's moral and spiritual foundation must now take place. One does not need to look very far to observe the damaging effect contemporary martial sport has had on the traditional principles of taekwondo. Standing ringside at tournaments, the spectator cannot help overhear verbal threats being exchanged between opponents prior to and during a match. These spectacles, while exciting to witness, tend to bring out a questionable character. Considering the honorable path of existence espoused by the Five Tenets of taekwondo, actions such as these are unbecoming a true martial artist and while they may be the exception in many cases, there is danger to the rule. Certainly, these contests have their place in testing one's technical ability in a confrontational environment. However, they should not be viewed as an end in themselves, but rather as a means of self-evaluation. Ideally, the diligent practice of taekwondo pits one against one's self in the ultimate contest of character. Therefore, if a student is truly drawn by the spirit of competition, they should then first try competing internally.

For example, waging a battle over obesity may be as arduous a task as anyone can imagine. In truth, many students enlist in the martial arts with just such a goal in mind. Setting measurable goals, a reasonable amount of weight loss tied to each successive belt level for instance, is not beyond the grasp of the modern day warrior. This "tournament" may prove as fierce as any contained by a sparring ring although the confidence and self-esteem generated by such a "win" cannot be cited by ribbons of any kind. Furthermore, training primarily for sport competition may tend to erode the defensive and spiritual value of taekwondo in a variety of ways. By instilling a "win at all

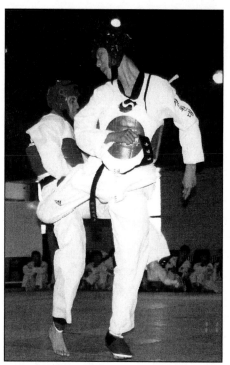

Korea traditionally has maintained the lead position in sport taekwondo.

costs" psychology in a student, the instructor is sending a mixed signal—on one hand preaching restraint against the use of excessive force during contact sparring, on the other teaching the doctrine of *il kyuk pil sul* or "first strike, swift and complete," in a defensive situation. This can harm the effectiveness of the techniques that are stamped in a practitioner's reactionary memory

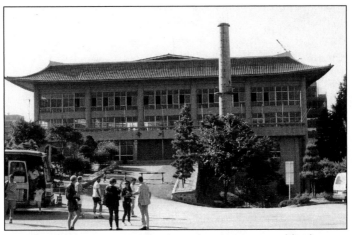

The Kukkiwon, center of taekwondo operations worldwide.

and ultimately breed confusion, causing the pupil to hesitate should a life threatening confrontation arise. Not unique to taekwondo, aikidoist Koichi Tohei takes aim at this issue when he observes, "The original intention of sports is to hold a contest of skills in accordance with rules and to enjoy the actual winning and losing. This is perfectly fine in these cases and in those martial arts that are describable as sports. The purpose of a real martial art, however, is quite different in that in both attack and defense we must always presuppose a genuine danger. Whatever

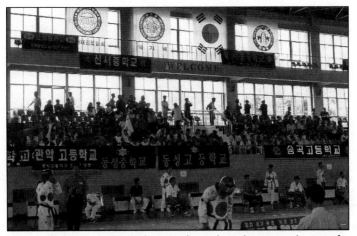

As well as being a martial art, taekwondo is the national sport of Korea. Here, a tournament is in progress at the Kukkiwon.

the opponent may do, it is useless to complain. We simply must act accordingly. Since our very lives are in danger, we must be prepared in both mind and body." In addition, there is a level of judgment and humility within the structure of a valid martial art one must indeed contend with. The teachings of the Buddhist monk Wonkwang, from which taekwondo's code of ethical behavior is derived, clearly encouraged the use of good judgment before harming any living thing. This guideline hints at the pacifist dimension of the martial arts; a domain in which the accomplished practitioner walks life's road armed with internal confidence, needing to prove his technical prowess to no one.

The fear also exists that taekwondo, the martial art, will be irrevocably diminished beyond recognition due to the attention and marketing currently being invested in what has become taekwondo, the combative Olympic sport. As a point of reference, one can see parallels of this trend dating back to the late 1800's in Jigoro Kano's creation of Kodokan judo. Sensing a decline in the popularity of jujutsu, Professor Kano, a noted educator, developed a sanitized version of the more aggressive Japanese martial art by removing techniques he felt were dangerous or out of step with the times. Originally intended as a means of inculcating moral principles and physical fitness in the Japanese population at large, the "gentle way" grew exponentially throughout the 1900's, eventually supplanting jujutsu as Japan's most pervasive martial discipline. With the cessation of hostilities at the conclusion of World War II, judo continued to pervade the Western world until reaching a high in 1964 with its inclusion in the Olympic games as a full medal sport—the only Asian martial art in history to bear this unique distinction at the time. Oddly enough, rather than attracting new practitioners to its ranks, recognition by the International Olympic Committee appears to have had the reverse effect on recruitment. Membership in what was once believed to be the world's most recognized martial art, began to subside. The current evolutionary phase judo now finds itself in is further complicated by the deterioration of various classical elements at the hands of those seeking to promote corporate sponsorships and media attention. While this course may be necessary for the sport to remain commercially viable in today's society, traditional rules and regulations that have gone untouched for decades are changing in favor of simplicity, linguistic advantage, and visual esthetics. Some in the martial arts community welcome these changes with open arms while others view them as a decrease in the standards set forth by the founder. In creating Kodokan judo, Jigoro Kano's original goal called for the gathering, filtering, and simplifying of the various combative styles of his day into one comprehensive syllabus. Ironically, with the simplification process coming full circle, certain philosophical elements have suffered.

As a case in point, judo, like aikido, relies on the yielding, blending, and redirection of an opponent's negative ki or aggressive energy to be effective. Being taught to win at any cost, however, flies in the face of this passive form of defense and other basic precepts as well. For example, it is now commonplace for the judo player to avoid being thrown by approaching the opponent in a crouched position rather than in the upright fighting stance found in the 1950's. In addition, the judo gi or jacket is often left open and untied with the belt worn low on the waist. This results not only in a sloppy appearance but has a negative effect on technique, translating into a defensive rather than an offensive spirit. Furthermore, efforts are underway to modernize the century old martial art by the introduction of a derivative style which replaces the traditional Japanese scoring terminology with a numerical point system and substitutes the familiar white uniform with one of contrasting color, more pleasing to the eye of the television camera.

The gradual decline of Kodokan judo from a martial art and sport rich with the philosophical overtones intended by its founder to its present diluted form, can in some ways be construed as a wake-up call to those who would unwittingly lead taekwondo down a similar path by encouraging competition at any cost. The danger exists that as dojangs heralding Olympic-style sparring as a main attraction proliferate, more and more tradition will be lost. This dilemma is made all the more poignant when one considers a statement made by martial arts instructor Jane Hallander in an article published by *Black Belt* titled, "Is Taekwondo a Sport or a Self-Defense System?" Acutely aware of the differences, Hallander warns, "There is more to taekwondo than just tournament competition. From kicks, to hand strikes, to throws, to joint locks, taekwondo possesses an array of defensive measures designed to thwart virtually any kind of attack. The most difficult part will not be learning these self-defense techniques, but finding a taekwondo instructor who still teaches them."

Having peeled away the superficial, competitive layer of taekwondo, what essential characteristics remain then to satisfy its mission as a modern day martial art? First, for any martial art to pass careful scrutiny, its syllabus must unquestionably contain legitimate defensive value. Taekwondo, in its traditional state, takes this requirement one step further by providing the practitioner with a full arsenal of offensive weapons in the shape of foot and hand techniques that compliment those of a primarily defensive nature. Many Asian fighting systems do not become effective until the aggressor has initiated an attack, thus leaving the defender in some danger. Conversely, the taekwondoist has at his disposal any number of techniques aimed at defusing a confrontational situation long

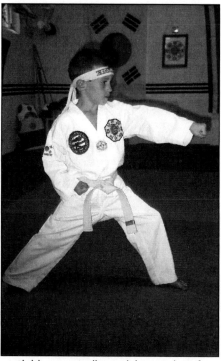

Children, as well as adults, can benefit greatly from the virtues of traditional taekwondo training.

before it has the opportunity to spin out of control. General Choi Hong Hi, the reputed founder of the term *taekwondo* and staunch defender regarding the traditional value of the art, clearly states that the Korean discipline contains over 3200 blocks, kicks, and strikes in addition to a multitude of leg sweeps, joint locks, and throws truly qualifying it as a complete form of self-defense. Still, certain factions persist in making false claims of

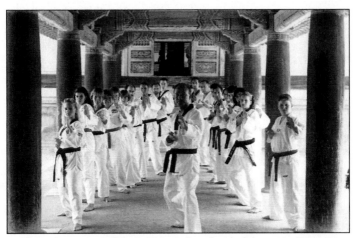

Grand Master Richard Chun and students of the United States Taekwondo Association at Pulguksa temple in Korea, demonstrating the two-hand knife block, a defensive technique found in traditional taekwondo.

inadequacy regarding the combat worthiness of taekwondo. This is not surprising coming from those trained exclusively in point-sparring where strikes are permitted only to areas protected by body armor and arm locks, sweeps, and throws are eliminated altogether.

In addition to a comprehensive collection of movements, taekwondo technique is further validated as a martial art through the watchful, unforgiving eye of careful scientific obser-

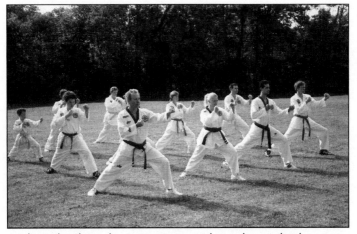

Traditional taekwondo training requires the student to develop strong basic technique.

vation. Newtonian physics teaches us that power equals mass multiplied by velocity as expressed in the formula:

$$P = mv$$

The taekwondoist trains diligently in drills aimed at refining the ability to explode into a target with lightning speed. Theoretically and in practice, this principle compensates for lack of body mass, allowing a person of lesser stature to dominate over a larger opponent. Again, we witness the stamp of scientific approval in the punching (jirugi) techniques of taekwondo where the law of conservation of energy rules. As the striking hand projects outward, twisting from the hip, the opposite hand is rotating back in forceful reciprocity on its return to the belt. Executed properly, this movement not only maintains the body's equilibrium but simultaneously results in an elbow strike (palkup chilki), a valuable asset in the practitioner's defensive inventory.

Yet another telling feature of a legitimate art is simplicity and elegance. In Chung Do Kwan taekwondo for instance, a system concentrating on the use of extreme power, the vast number of techniques available to the student are pared down to a bare minimum with a strong emphasis placed on flawless form and focus. The strikes used are executed at maximum force without hesitation or restraint. Again, we see the simple strategy of quality over quantity in action. Likewise, while it may appear strange to some, the martial artist sees majesty in a well-executed block or strike. The essence and esthetic beauty of taekwondo is often reflected in the sublime performance of poom-se, a method by which technique can be dynamically practiced to perfection. The articulation of the hands in a double middle knife block (dool sonnal momtang maggi), the graceful arc traced through the air of a crescent kick (pyojok chagi), the sharp linear path of a reverse punch (bandae jirugi), all comply with the definition of art-in-motion. Parallels can be drawn to dance, a similar art of movement that satisfies the need for the human spirit to assert itself in space.

Moreover, longevity and depth of technique are further indicators of an art's veracity. While it is not required that a martial discipline be ancient to qualify as traditional, it can be helpful. Today, we find techniques that served the Hwarang in seventh century Silla being employed in modern day taekwondo. Theoretically, experienced warriors returning from battle would proudly demonstrate the kicks, blocks, and strikes relied upon to survive for the benefit of eager recruits who, in turn, would mimic them in hopes of being equally triumphant. In this way the native arts of kwonbop, taekkyon, and subahk were handed down from generation to generation. However, simply because something has been repeated over the centuries does not necessarily make it better. Just as in Darwin's *Origin of the Species* concerning evolution, certain superfluous techniques of dubious value have, in all likelihood, been cast away over time leaving only those of absolute necessity. By the same token, additions have been made to the preexisting arsenal of techniques in an effort to offset radical advances in technology. A worthy example of this may be the development and inclusion of specific tactics aimed at defending against the use of hand-held firearms. This ebb and flow of technique is employed in preserving economy of form, an essential ingredient common to all artful endeavors. Viewed from a practical standpoint, economy of form results in an elegant system of defensive techniques that the martial artist can reflexively call upon at a moment's notice without confusion or hesitation.

Even though the movements of taekwondo have been mapped out in precise detail, as with any art, room remains for self-expression. A casual look at the many technical volumes available on the subject will, through the use of charts and illustrations, accurately reveal the exact angular composition of a stance, the alignment of kicks and strikes, and the correct movements within a given form. However, since no two human beings are physically identical, this information will be digested and executed uniquely. Therefore, while the gifted athlete may find these techniques simple to perform, there is little doubt that even the most awkward among us can benefit greatly from the balance and poise instilled by the diligent practice of taekwondo. After countless repetitions of a particular poom-se for instance, the practitioner cannot help but exhibit a renewed sense of confidence in his body's ability to move freely through the spatial plane while constantly redefining these motions with highlights of a highly personal nature. Clearly, as we grow older, whether it be a function of the body's natural deterioration, or the fear and embarrassment associated with a seemingly nonsensical expression of locomotion, the majority of us stop moving simply for the fun of it. Who is to say that age must curtail the enjoyment of such overt movement? Certainly it can be said that popular dance and some forms of sport fulfill this primordial need. Still, just as there are those who require more than an aerobics class to feel physically satisfied, there are those who look for a deeper meaning from movement. Isn't it odd that it may take a martial art, a discipline originally intended for use on the field of battle, to reawaken the sense of movement within us and act in a spiritually therapeutic manner? This harmony that exists between traditional structure and expressive freedom further verifies the value of taekwondo as a traditional martial art.

Perhaps the greatest indicator of taekwondo's artistic contribution to the fulfillment of the individual is the emphasis placed on cultivating the mind, body, and soul. This holistic approach, as described in a previous chapter, lies at the very core of the discipline's ideology. The Hwarang, who not only practiced the martial arts, but also fed their mind and spirit with the study of music, poetry, and Confucian philosophy, exemplified this time-honored tradition. Consequently, whereas the contemporary athlete may concentrate primarily on bodybuilding and strategies specific to a given sport, the modern day warrior reverently trains not only in the physical aspects of taekwondo, but also seeks to bolster valuable mental and spiritual capabilities through studies in Asian history and ki development.

In the final analysis, there should be little question regarding taekwondo's validity as a martial art. However, it would be just as irresponsible to simply dismiss its popularity as a modern, combative sport. Certainly, it is this very popularity that has catapulted taekwondo into the Olympic arena, and the collective consciousness of the world at large. But, as Grand Master Sang Kyu Shim points out, "The martial arts are not mere sport, despite a superficial resemblance between the two. Some enthusiasts would like to see the martial arts included in Olympic competitions. This is contrary to the nature and spirit of the martial arts. Commendable as the Olympics may be as a form of international competition, they are not a way of life, as the martial arts, in their true sense are." Thus, we are reminded that, by its very nature, competitive sport assumes there will always be a winner and a loser, a victor and a vanquished. From a youthful age we, as a society, are taught, "it doesn't matter if you win or lose, it's how you play the game." In contrast, we reward our winning athletes with multi-million dollar contracts and product endorsement agreements with little or no attention given to the "losers." One wonders if this is a worthy method of instilling a sense of virtue in our adolescent or adult population. With this in mind, students need to be periodically reminded that even though testing one's abilities in the ring at first appears to be an exciting proposition, it does not mirror the true philosophical essence of taekwondo.

Therefore, it is essential that students be made aware of the distinction between martial art and martial sport early on so that they may choose wisely in their selection of a dojang that will meet their established goals. To many, this distinction will be a matter of perception. As a case in point, taekwondo may represent nothing more than a substitute for bowling or soccer practice. To these individuals who wish no more from the martial arts other than social interaction and a means of physical fitness, the sportive experience may prove both rewarding and exhilarating. On the other hand, those with different expectations may choose to delve deeper into the spiritual aspects surrounding taekwondo, requiring a greater commitment on the part of the practitioner. But in the end, after much debate and controversy, it is clear that taekwondo the martial art, replete with its tradition and philosophy, must ultimately learn to coexist with taekwondo, the martial sport, if either are to continue living.

CHAPTER 16

Beyond Black Belt: Staying the Course

Climbing the ladder to the black belt is an experience filled with emotions that span the entire spectrum of the human condition. Situations arise that incite otherwise meek women to forcefully assert themselves and grown men to cry. Cycles are created mirroring the very nature of life itself. Although unclear to the novice at the time, these internal conflicts are sure indicators that the ideological underpinnings of taekwondo are beginning to penetrate. Mercurial shifts in behavior are not unusual given the level of personal commitment required in attaining the greatest symbolic privilege taekwondo has to offer. Technical prowess in the Korean martial arts does not come easy and demands a great deal of time and effort to perfect. So much, in fact, that many newcomers find it difficult, if not impossible, to acquire the high level of proficiency necessary to earn the coveted black belt. Not surprisingly, current statistical evidence demonstrates that only one in every fifty practitioners contending for this prize ultimately fulfills the terms required to achieve it. Being aware of this ratio, the taekwondoist should be all the more appreciative of this accomplishment when it is finally realized. Once attained however, the martial artist gradually awakens to the notion that this is merely a point of departure—the first step on a road that, if traveled with diligence, will never see an end.

Aside from its value as denoting a rank in a system of colored belts, the black belt itself should be viewed primarily as a token of the martial artist's growing maturity, not simply in chronological terms, but in depth of knowledge and technical ability. Ignorance of martial arts hierarchy generally compels one to believe that receiving a black belt in a given discipline represents the final reward in a lengthy round of training sessions; a fabric diploma awarded at the completion of a course in self-

159

defense. In reality, however, the black belt represents a different type of document. It is a birth certificate of sorts that announces that the holder is born and, like a newborn yearning to explore, thirsts to expand on the techniques learned as a colored belt. Some practitioners restrict their training to the first dan level, never allowing themselves the benefits inherent in reaching full maturity. Not surprisingly, the attrition rate in the martial arts increases proportionally as one rises through the dan grades.

Why is this? Why, after investing heavily in years of intense training, would the black belt student, regardless of age, abandon the skills earned in so worthy a quest? Clearly, as with any physical activity of this nature, any number of excuses can be offered for the pupil's misguided desire to cease training. Author, school owner, and instructor, John Graden, in an article published by *Inside Taekwondo* magazine, describes why he feels students become bored with their martial arts training. Lack of discernible progress, goals, recognition, and enthusiasm in the dojang environment, he states, all contribute greatly to the malaise sometimes experienced by the black belt student. For instance, after becoming accustomed to routinely testing every few months, the black belt now faces a period of years before a formal challenge of skill is required according to curriculum. This alone can lead to an attitude marred by complacency. Many school instructors confront this issue by holding intermediate tests within the dan level, thus pushing the student to maintain a high level of technical excellence. This methodology serves the dual purpose of setting measurable goals that act as milestones on the road to the next dan rank while at the same time satisfying the acquired need to develop new and exciting techniques. Likewise, being recognized by an observant instructor for achievements large and small can have a direct result on the black belt student's sense of self-esteem, both in and out of the dojang. This holds especially true for the mature black belt, earnestly trying to become proficient in an art that requires a sometimes overwhelming amount of mental and physical discipline.

On the other hand, many departing students sincerely view their ascension to black belt as a completion of their training and either dabble in yet another martial art or, if originally concerned with health issues, switch to a similar form of activity geared towards physical fitness. In the case of the former, it is generally suggested that a pupil continue practicing taekwondo, or any martial art for that matter, for a period of not less than eight years before cross training. As for the latter, the potential for physical fitness is greatly enhanced at the black belt level due to an increase of expectations based on dojang curriculum. It fact, it has been determined that following a disciplined martial arts fitness program will burn more calories in a given timeframe than will any other form of exercise. However, as with any endeavor of this sort, there are the more obvious issues such as demands on available time, work-related matters, or family obligations. If resolved, solutions to these problems may ultimately have a positive bearing on salvaging the pupil's future training. But if not these reasons, what other possible objections could the disenchanted black belt raise in defense of their departure? Probably the most malignant of all excuses and one that is neither easy to identify nor pleasant to admit, is a profound loss of the underlying motivation that had caused the student to

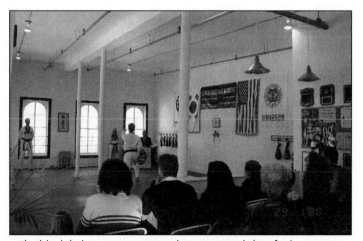

The black belt test is an extremely serious and dignified occasion.

commence training in the first place.

In past chapters, we have cited many of the overt reasons that may initially draw an individual to the martial arts. These include a desire to study self-defense, become physically fit, and to practice a traditional, ritualistic discipline devoid of religious dogma. Suffice it to say that whatever the rationale behind enrollment, almost without fail a catharsis takes place following the first few training sessions that reaches to the very core of the student's spiritual domain. Subsequently, the secret to remaining motivated in the martial arts lies in the enlightenment that results from allowing this newly acquired passion to burn brightly, unhindered by excessive self-criticism or activities that can mask one of the true intentions of taekwondo training—confidence leading to self-determination and thus, self-fulfillment. Those who aspire to the black belt continue to carry this internal flame within themselves, unextinguished over the years. Admittedly, it is unrealistic to expect one to remain in a constant state of emotional equilibrium day after day. Rather, it is more likely that the physical and mental resilience needed to practice taekwondo will mimic the student's daily mood swings. A competent instructor may sense the temporary dimming of this flame and attempt to rekindle it through compassion and encouragement. Others, more concerned with loss of income should the student turn his back on the martial arts, will resort to intimidation and manipulation in a flawed attempt at retention. Consequently, much of what makes the taekwondoist a successful martial artist is not the invasive measures of a heavy-handed master, but the personal expression of a student's passion through perseverance, diligence, loyalty to the art, and trust in the instincts of a forthright instructor.

Those of us who wholeheartedly embrace the martial arts as a way of life seldom need to be reminded of the intensity with which this passion burns. Instead, we eagerly look to fulfill the opportunities that rank and tenure brings. While these opportunities come in a variety of shapes and sizes, clearly one of the most noble is the act of instructing. Teaching is an art and, as such, may not befit the temperament and talents of every black belt. Nor can a practitioner automatically be expected to assume command of a class based purely on superior rank. However, there is no reason why the black belt should not begin, at the first dan level, to develop the fundamental skills required to transmit the gift of taekwondo along to other worthy candidates. Moreover, a segment of students will naturally aspire to become

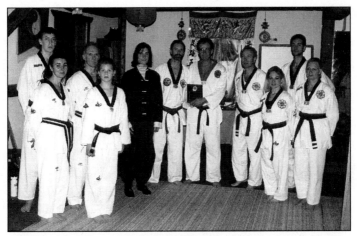

The black belt has earned respect through hard training and holds an esteemed position in a school's hierarchy.

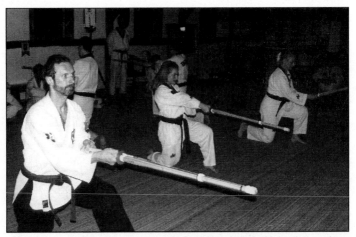

Weapons training usually reserved for black belt holders due to their elevated level of self-control.

instructors while others may choose to practice their art within themselves. Regardless, the black belt student should, at minimum, be expected to teach by example.

Even though a task of this magnitude may at first appear simple, in truth it is difficult at best, given the temptations and moral breakdown evident in modern society. This is not to suggest that the actions of the martial artist are expected to approach messianic proportions. On the contrary, in setting an example for society, the black belt must first begin by exhibiting humility. As we have seen, the general public sometimes mistakenly ascribes superhuman powers to the martial artist. Therefore, it is the responsibility of the black belt not to permit this belief to manifest itself in unrestrained pride or aggression. Speaking parenthetically from Zen philosophy, usually those that have the least to say, speak the most. On yet another level, color belt students constantly look to their black belt colleagues for direction and methods to improve their own techniques. What better way, then, to nurture teaching ability than to strive for one's own personal perfection as an example to others. In light of this, it is mandatory that the black belt be aware of the part they play in acting as a role model to others, not only in the dojang, but outside as well. Appraisal and refinement of one's character is a basic principle that touches the very heart of modern day taekwondo training.

Yet another step in the maturation process of the black belt is the transition from a predominately physical outlook on the martial arts to one of philosophical awareness. Most color belts, eager to be informed and enlightened by the ideological precepts of Eastern philosophy that underscore traditional taekwondo, are understandably more concerned with expanding their technical horizons. Concepts regarding ki development and the relationship between meditation and religion in the martial arts can potentially breed confusion and are often outside the scope of those less experienced in the martial way. Consequently, a vast majority of instructors do not even begin discussing these matters with their students until black belt level, if at all. In many ways this is unfortunate given the fertile soil fresh minds offer in accepting the new and the different. However, by the time the black belt is awarded, the practitioner's mind should be sufficiently fit and open to digest some of the more esoteric concepts that nurture the harmony between mind, body, and soul. An acceptance of change, as seen in the shifting patterns of the Um/Yang and the I Ching, coupled with a deep appreciation for the natural order of the universe, can be viewed as indicators of the martial artist's expanding bank of wisdom.

Taekwondo, being the action philosophy that it is, cannot function correctly as an effective means of self-defense without a strong physical foundation supporting these spiritual and intellectual elements. Shortly after receiving the black belt then, the taekwondoist should expect to experience yet another period of rapid growth as the skills transmitted from instructor to pupil during the color belt years are polished. This honing process requires that the adherent perform the basic techniques with great care and deliberation, placing each motion beneath the virtual lens of a microscope and dissecting it into its various dynamic components. The hands should always be set, the blocks exaggerated, and the stances sturdy and balanced yet not grossly overstated. Strikes should be backed by the explosive power of ki and executed in a strong, linear, or circular fashion while never reaching beyond the intended target area. By now, the student should possess the requisite flexibility and focus, that magical combination of power, speed, and concentration needed to place a kick at any desired vital point on the human anatomy. Moreover, possessed with a confidence that can only be gained through countless repetitions of poom-se, the black belt student will be pleased to discover a fluidity of movement marking the union of the physical being and the meditative state of mind. Those with an eye for such qualities and distinctions will recognize this union for what it truly is—a verification of the art in taekwondo.

As any student who has trained in the martial arts for a number of years can attest, the demons of doubt and discouragement lie in wait at every turn. Consequently, those elite few who eventually earn the black belt have every reason to bathe in the glory of their achievement. Often there is a certain pride that accompanies human accomplishment of this magnitude. Therefore, while it is natural for the student to speak openly of the passion he feels towards taekwondo, he must never act in an arrogant or threatening manner, but hold his technical gifts in abeyance until such time when they are needed. The black belt must accept the awesome powers bestowed by his instructors with both humility and respect. Furthermore, the pupil, realizing that he continues to be a novice even at the first dan level, must remain humble and open to accepting new and advanced techniques. In some cases, however, vanity can cloud one's ability to accept new ideas.

Take for instance the tale of the old Japanese Zen master

who was engaged in conversation with a student as related by Peter Lewis in his book, *The Martial Arts: Origin, Philosophy, Practice*:

> *The student chatted on and on, full of his own opinions and ideas. He described to the master everything he knew about Zen, trying to impress the old man with his great knowledge. The master sat and listened patiently, then suggested that they take some tea. The student held out his cup dutifully and the master began to pour. The tea came to the top of the cup, but still the master kept on pouring. The tea overflowed but still the master kept on. The student unable to contain himself, pointed out that no more tea would go into the cup. The master looked up and said "Like this cup you are full of your own desires and ambitions. How then can I show you Zen unless you first empty your cup?"*

Clearly, in keeping with the Zen doctrine of "beginner's mind" as discussed earlier, the student must set aside previously established opinions and preconceptions, and leave them at the threshold of the dojang.

Most importantly, the black belt must never lose sight of the future. After coming to grips with the qualifications and expectations commensurate with rank, the first dan must set his sights on advanced levels of proficiency and responsibility in the martial arts. Training in traditional weapons such as the *nunchaku* (*song jul kwon*), the *bo* staff (*jung bong*), and the bamboo sword (*jook do*), are often best left for introduction at the black belt level due to the advanced level of respect necessary for their use coupled with the student's rapidly expanding ability of self-control. In conjunction with these skills, the black belt will begin to learn the dramatic aerial kicks unique to the art of taekwondo. Likewise, on a strategic plain, the measurable goals set in attaining the colored belts must be equally applied to advancement through the dan grades. Poom-se and physical technique become increasingly difficult, demanding more commitment and focus by the black belt. More to the point, the martial artist cannot be excused from framing a program geared to achieve predetermined results simply because the time span between promotion examinations is prolonged. Additionally, since self-determination plays such an integral part in the philosophy of taekwondo, the black belt must constantly strive to uncover methods that will aid in steering a unique course through life—a path unaffected by the whims and desires of those concerned exclusively with their own selfish gain and welfare. This is not to say that the adherent must become insensitive to the needs of others. On the contrary, benevolence and compassion are key traits of the black belt and must be continually cultivated and constantly practiced.

As we have seen, becoming a black belt in taekwondo, or any martial art for that matter, requires focus, determination, and perseverance. But one must never underestimate the patience demanded in the process. Just as it takes centuries for a rushing river to cut a great canyon, the transformation from the ordinary to an exemplary individual takes time. But, once the color belt crosses the threshold to black belt, certain intangible dynamics are revealed. As an example, a centering takes place whereby correct posture becomes the norm and the body appears relaxed and settled. Likewise, at work or in school, the black belt can maintain concentration for longer periods of time. Furthermore, friends and neighbors are often surprised at the unconditional courtesy afforded them and will comment in return on the practitioner's healthy appearance. And lastly, the positive demeanor exuded by a person confident in the fact that they can defend themselves against adversity is eclipsed only by the triumphs they leave in their wake. Even though these changes may seem inconsequential to others less concerned with self-improvement, they are monumental to the martial artist who, having nurtured these attributes over the years, can now finally begin to reap their benefits. Accompanied by the pride, honor and satisfaction that comes with dan rank, the black belt will persevere while rapidly growing secure in the knowledge that the never-ending journey on the road to advancement in taekwondo is certain to hold many undiscovered rewards.

CHAPTER 17

An Action Philosophy

Imagine for a moment what the world would be like today if the incandescent lamp had remained only a spark in the mind of Thomas Alva Edison. Consider how empty America's roadways would be were it not for a man named Henry Ford who managed to mass-produce an affordable mode of transportation. These marvelous inventions, along with their profound effects on mankind, have one thing in common—they were born as a direct result of their creators putting thought into action.

The road to accomplishment is littered with the good intentions of those who tragically have permitted their hopes to remain locked in their head. Instead of implementing their plans, they hold them prisoner, only to be released at some later date as regretful reminders of the way things might have been. They enviously admire the success of their peers, and often wonder just what chemistry brought about their good fortune. Still others suffer the jealousy and despair that go hand in hand with such negative emotions. Each one of us, at one time or another, has had a unique idea that could in some way potentially pose a benefit to humanity. Yet, even with these bursts of imagination tugging at the creative fibers of the soul, it is difficult to admit that we hold the power to significantly change our life, and the lives of those around us, with only a single thought put into motion. Perhaps one reason for this is that the skills necessary to animate our dreams are not readily accessible to the vast majority of us. Add to this the fact that the requisite attributes of courage and perseverance, so essential to any personal venture, are not universally developed and we begin to see why so many of us reside in a creative netherland hovering between self-fulfillment and endless frustration.

One needs only to visit the shelves of a local bookstore to realize that there is no limit to the amount of written material on the subject of self-improvement. Motivational speakers and business consultants abound in today's highly charged, economically driven environment. While their methods and suggestions may set the stage for a plan of action, they are fundamentally flawed in that they cannot genuinely instill the confidence necessary to fulfill this action. It takes more than clever marketing phrases and insincere smiles to nurture the discipline, integrity, and indomitable spirit necessary to become worthy of today's cultural challenges. In truth, a system of holistic development aimed at cultivating the individual's internal resolve, physical stamina, spiritual awareness, and mental acuity is what ultimately is required. Clearly, there are a number of routes one can take in acquiring these elusive characteristics, but none so thorough as the martial arts. If approached in a traditional manner, taekwondo, in particular, has the ability to satisfy the needs of the modern day warrior in facing the trials and tribulations of daily life. Again the question arises: How can an ancient system of potentially lethal kicks and punches be expected to reinforce, or in some cases replace, the socially accepted academic, religious, and fitness programs in cultivating a positive, action-based outlook toward life? In answering this question, we must first determine just what it is that makes taekwondo such a motivating force and examine whether these elements can truly act as a legitimate alternative to the self-improvement systems that are currently in place.

To begin with, we can say that taekwondo is an action philosophy because its roots lie in the vigorous implementation of its various techniques, not simply in a sterile dissertation of how they should be accomplished. In truth, many instructors fall prey to the mistake of over verbalizing a set of movements rather than allowing the muscles to learn by experiencing the motion. Dave Lowry in *Black Belt* magazine points out that, "The training process in most martial arts is certainly intellectual to some extent. But the primary method of learning is for the body to absorb and understand." He goes on to say, "The body learns much differently than the mind. We can sit and read about a front kick, we can ask our seniors about it, and we can watch videotapes of it. We may come to be experts in all the information available about the kick, but until our body can actually perform it, we don't understand it at all." By its very nature, proficiency in taekwondo requires that the practitioner repeat a technique thousands of times before he can truly claim it as his own. As we have seen, this concept is equally valid for sparring and basics as it is for poom-se practice. Furthermore, attempting to explain the dynamic elements involved in the proper execution of a roundhouse kick without doing it is tantamount to describing the color red to a sightless person. As Mr. Lowry puts it, "I can tell you how an apple tastes, but to experience it, you have to taste it yourself." Therefore, no amount of book study, no matter how descriptive or correct, can take the place of diligent, physical practice in the dojang. Certainly, as humans we must allow for inconsistencies in our training schedule. There will be times when a strenuous workout will be the least attractive part of the practitioner's day regardless of their love for taekwondo. However, it is times such as these that the true martial artist must rise to the occasion and train harder, lest they become awash in a wave of complacency.

On yet another level, the taekwondoist should realize that action can present itself in a variety of ways. In a confrontational situation with an assailant for instance, physical action will be required even if it is negative action in the form of passive behavior. As an example, through the use of strategic techniques learned in the dojang, the martial artist will often feign retreat in an attempt to observe the offensive maneuvers of the opponent while simultaneously formulating an effective counterattack. This approach is likened to the ancient Taoist philosophical paradox of action manifesting itself through inaction. Or, similar to the selfless characteristics of water as portrayed in *Poom-se Taegeuk Yook Jang,* allowing an event to take its course without intervention can be construed as a form of action in and of itself. Signified by the principle of *gam* that lies within the eight trigrams of the *palgwe,* Taegeuk Yook Jang further illustrates this philosophy by teaching us that water never loses its characteristics of consistency and flow. If a stream in its travel encounters an obstacle, it will continue unhindered around it, eventually wearing it down. The passive action of water, therefore, naturally avoids resistance and symbolizes the tolerance, consistency, and natural integrity we must demonstrate as martial artists if we are to endure life's adversities.

Sitting meditation also teaches us much regarding the passive nature of action. To the uneducated observer, a practitioner seated in *seiza* posture would appear to be the epitome of inaction—a serene human form in a state of total relaxation. However, being familiar with the process, nothing could be further from the truth. As we have come to see, meditation in its various iterations can be demanding work. Maintaining correct body alignment, counting breaths, or merely visualizing a desired scenario requires a great deal of concentration and effort on the part of the meditator and again demonstrates the principle of action residing at the core of apparent inaction. In a similar situation, the cultivation and development of internal ki energy through

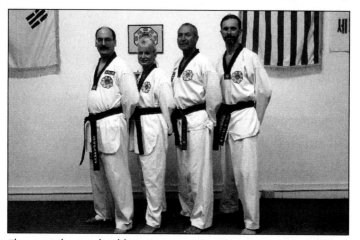

The martial artist should strive to maintain an active, positive attitude both inside and outside the dojang.

the use of specialized breathing methods calls for an equally concerted effort. In fact, if done correctly, the perspiration culled from such labor can be compared with the sweat generated by a decathlon runner, thus confirming the actively intense nature of its practice.

This dichotomy of apparent inaction as opposed to the direct application of action can easily be found in all facets of taekwondo. In yet another example of the action philosophy, forward-thinking moral judgment can be seen in an energetic belief of taekwondo's five tenets—courtesy, integrity, perseverance, self-control, and indomitable spirit. Each of these virtues requires that the martial artist act on them in some altruistic manner. Everyday we are given opportunities to exemplify these ideals. The simple act of holding a door open for an elderly person or making a determined effort to continue a particularly difficult task is a manifestation of the action-based philosophy. Moreover, by routinely reciting the ten ethical principles at the culmination of a training session, the taekwondoist further commits to the qualities of this action philosophy, in thought and deed, on a daily level. What good could simple acts of courtesy as expressed by a single individual have on the world at large? In answer to this, the native Korean philosophy, "Su Shin Je Ga Chi Guk Pyong Chun Fa" states, "Peace within myself brings peace within the family. Peace in the family brings peace in the community. Peace in the community brings peace in the country. " And finally, "Peace in the country brings peace in the world." If one were to delve even deeper into Asian history, he would find a direct correlation between these words and those of the great Eastern philosopher, Confucius, when he wrote, "If there is righteousness in the heart, there will be beauty in the character. If there is beauty in the character, there will be harmony in the home. If there is harmony in the home, there will be order in the nation. If there is order in the nation, there will be peace in the world." Like ripples on a pond, benevolent deeds radiate outward.

Further, by accepting a belt of any color, the practitioner assumes the unique role of an exemplary individual in the process of nurturing leadership skills. Society exhibits a propensity for flocking to the person who possesses focus and determination. These elements, in conjunction with confidence and a measure of common sense, label a man or woman as a natural leader. Leadership however, is a hollow virtue without the ability to transform concept into reality. Leadership demands action.

The responsible implementation of action however, does not come without its hazards. Once a concept is put into motion and gains momentum, it tends to take on a life of its own. Subsequently, it is essential that we examine the potential outcome of our actions carefully before executing them. Do they fit the criteria set forth under the martial artist's code of honor? What long-term effects will they have on those most affected?

Are they justified? Searching back through Korean history, we see that the tiny kingdom of Silla, known for its valor and courage, practiced great forbearance and compassion even in its reach for territorial triumph. During the first century A.D., under the reign of King P'a-sa, Silla began to actively expand its borders. Said to be a great administrator and kind conqueror, the monarch ruled wisely by exerting action in a benign manner to the benefit of his many new subjects. Unlike many of his counterparts, the king provided for the vanquished, and was concerned for their welfare. Since we, as taekwondoists, often look to Sillian and thus Hwarang-do ethical standards as a template for modern day living, the actions of numerous Korean rulers and military men who eventually unified the country should be used as a model for our own present day actions.

On a more contemporary level, however, everyone is familiar with the phrase, "actions speak louder than words." This is especially true of the martial artist who routinely practices restraint and humility over excess and pride. Making promises that one does not intend to keep or bragging endlessly regarding one's accomplishments is clearly not in keeping with the martial way. It is natural for an individual to harbor dreams and aspirations that occasionally bubbles over in a froth of enthusiasm. Often these hopes do not come to fruition even though they are expressed with the utmost sincerity. Judging from their source, these ambitions are frequently not based on irresponsibility, but fraught with the greatest desire to succeed and must be separated from those of sinister intent. The pure of heart will recognize this difference in motive as a reflection of their own personal endeavors and will react accordingly. Armed with this knowledge, the practitioner must realize that actions of any order are powerful entities laden with consequence and deserving of vigilant and prudent forethought.

Therefore, we find that a real possibility exists for the martial arts to act as an overriding influence and alternative partner to the current social structures at large, as posited earlier, in determining an action based philosophy. However, one must test the feasibility of this program in supporting these institutions according to their individual need. We find that devout faith in the church will doubtless instill hope in the believer and act as fuel for the soul. Conversely, a disciplined routine of exercise will improve and tone the body, offering enhanced health and a sense of physical pride. Likewise, the academic pursuit of a given topic within a proper scholastic environment will satisfy the thirst for knowledge. But where, we ask, is the confluence between the three? At what point do the spiritual, physical, and intellectual meet in a harmonious, holistic blend? Upon closer examination we realize that in cultivating an action philosophy, it is important that we as human beings feel vested with spiritual enlightenment, physical strength, and intellectual skill. But, like a three-legged stool, none of these can successfully exist on their own if we are to be truly fulfilled. Therefore, in looking to the martial arts as a binding force, we discover that a number of methods exist within the framework of taekwondo for satisfying the need to experience all three of these virtues both singularly and in concert through a program of diligent and sincere practice.

Clearly, the martial artist is the sum of many parts, action not being the least of them. As a function of this, the modern day warrior must display courageous behavior at all times, and not become mired down in desperation as a result of adversity. This is not to say that decisions should be clouded by insensitivity. On the contrary, actions should be based upon a thorough understanding of the real issues at hand and then, once arrived at, acted on decisively. However, action must also be tempered with judgment. Just as judgment must spring from wisdom, wisdom (at least as it applies to taekwondo), can ultimately be gained from a thoughtful pursuit of the ethical and spiritual principles handed down over the centuries by kings, warriors, monks, and fellow martial artists who have traditionally, and with sincerity, subscribed to a philosophy of action.

CHAPTER 18

Do: A Way of Life

Do. Pronounced "doe," this simple, two-lettered syllable symbolizes the spiritual, intellectual, and ethical dimensions manifest in the traditional Korean martial art of taekwondo. It is the essence and standard against which all practical and theoretical technique is measured. Literally translated, it is the "Way" or "Path" every martial artist must travel. It is the level we must attain and the ideal we embrace. It is a work constantly in progress. Sang Kyu Shim put this journey in perspective when he wrote, "One must not confuse the skills of living with the way of living. The martial arts point the way while providing the skills to follow the Way. This is the road to creative change, a road of encounter and discovery; it is the road of a million miles that begins with the first step."

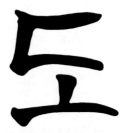

The Hangul representation of do.

To underestimate the significance of do due to its grammatical positioning within the root word taekwondo, is to admit to a profound ignorance in this diverse, holistic discipline. To subtract this suffix is to remove the heart and soul of the art, transforming it instead into a mere pugilistic pursuit, a physical skill rather than an organic philosophy complete with a ritualized set of moral principles. Furthermore, while it is true that the term taekwondo itself is only a few decades old, the fact remains that the art we know today draws these principles from a mixture of traditional fighting styles rooted deep in Korean history. Still, there are those who assert that taekwondo has no true heritage, that it is nothing more than a competitive sport—a bastard child of Japanese karate or Chinese gongfu. These are the few who are unwilling to see value in the Way.

The contemporary concept of do partially stems from a

desire expressed by noted masters of the past to transform their traditional martial skills, no longer as relevant in times of peace, into martial ways. Simply put, a martial way distinguishes itself from a fighting art in that the ultimate goal is not necessarily one of combat preparedness so much as it is a means to achieve personal excellence through a practice of the martial arts accompanied by their implied codes of honor. By way of example, taekwondo, tang soo do, karatedo, aikido and judo are all offspring of fighting systems used mainly for the purpose of subduing an adversary in battle and expanded upon by their innovators in modern times to include a road map for ethical living. Men such as General Choi Hong Hi, Hwang Kee, Gichen Funakoshi, Morihei Ueshiba and Jigoro Kano appreciated the value of elevating their native defensive skills into usable disciplines intended to instill confidence and morality in society at large. Consequently, tens of millions of practitioners worldwide study some form of martial art in an effort to fortify their physical, mental, and spiritual capabilities while actively becoming proficient in a style of self-defense.

But this is not the first mention we find in Asian history regarding do as an enlightened path to moral behavior. Perhaps the oldest and most noted writings on the subject can be traced to Lao Tzu, philosopher and author of the *Tao Teh Ching* or the "Way of Virtue." Transcribed sometime during the fourth century B.C., it is the centerpiece of Taoist tradition. Originally, it was promoted as a poetic treatise on the art of politics, government, and virtue and was intended to bring harmony between warring factions during a particularly turbulent period in Chinese history. This desire is clearly stated by the author in verse number 30 where he states:

> *After you have attained your purpose, You must not parade your success, You must not boast of your ability, You must not feel proud, You must rather regret that you had not been able to prevent the war. You must never think of conquering others by force. For to be over-developed is to hasten decay. And this is against tao, And what is against tao will soon cease to be.*

Echoes of this advice ring down through the centuries and find a sympathetic ear even today in taekwondo philosophy. For example, the martial artist is often exhorted to recall that "the only good fight is the one that is never fought," bringing to mind the words of the ancient Taoist sage. Likewise, we are reminded to "use good judgment in battle" and to "display humility" at all times, proving further that these verses stand the test of time within the freedoms of our own modern civilization.

Taoism and its reliance on the Way remains a cornerstone of Eastern thought to this day and has given rise to what is perhaps one of the most recognized icons of all time, the Yin/Yang.

This symbol is composed of two tear-shaped elements cir-

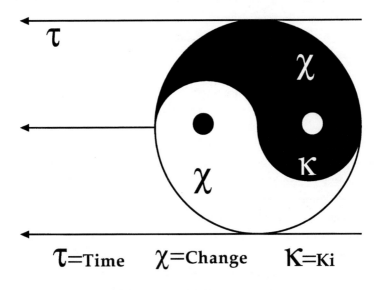

τ=Time χ=Change   K=Ki

The Spiral Nature of the Yin/Yang.

cling one another. Nestled in the lobe of each is a representative sample of its mate. On a three-dimensional level, this elementary circle can be extrapolated into two, discreet orbiting polarities thus giving rise to a spiral, satisfying both the cyclical and linear natures of life as we travel through time. The Yin/Yang, furthermore, acts as a metaphor for the duality of opposites, the struggle between two opposing forces to exist in a state of equilibrium. Moreover, it embraces a belief in constant change as a central dynamic of do in daily living. Even though certain characteristics of this symbol are altered in both the Korean (Um/Yang) and Japanese (In/Yo) cultures, the underlying principles inherent in its design remain the same. Depicted in its simplicity is the never-ending harmony that exists between two unlike forces; forces such as light and dark, soft and hard, right and left, goodness and evil, and night and day. This harmonic resolution rests on the fact that, rather than negating one another, these contradictions are supportive in their oneness. Um is considered the passive, receptive polarity while Yang can be thought of as the assertive or active partner. Dividing them, is a high energy, sine-curve boundary line. Rather than remaining in a static state, this division vibrates kinetically with ki, the vital life force.

Even though we are familiar with ki from a previous chapter, it is worthwhile noting Grand Master Richard Chun's definition as it applies to the duality of opposites. Here he states, "Ki is the cosmic ocean in which everything exists. It is kept in balance by the Um/Yang working in rhythm. It is at its best when it flows freely, neither too active nor too passive, but in perfect harmonic balance." Taking a utilitarian approach to the basic theme underscoring the Um/Yang can have a significant effect on the practical application of taekwondo technique in general. For no matter where we turn in following the natural order of the Way, we are constantly reminded of the simple wisdom inherent in this unique symbol. For example, the very basis of martial arts movement now and in the past can be traced to the observation and mimicry of nature. Many of the more advanced strikes and stances such as tiger mouth strike (*kumsohn*) and cat stance (*poom sogi*), derive their very names from the defensive tactics seen in the animal kingdom. Likewise, the method of wrist rotation found in the execution of the middle punch (*momtang jirugi*) while in horseback stance (*jachoom sogi*), replicates the revolution of the planets as described in the physics of celestial mechanics. Furthermore, poom-se, the choreographed forms that stand as a central pillar of traditional taekwondo, are rich in an abundance of natural metaphor. Borrowing heavily from the *I Ching*, these essential patterns draw their philosophical individualism from the palgwe whose eight sets of trigrams represent nature in its fullness. The virtues of thunder, wind, water, fire, and earth are all in evidence as the practitioner learns to overcome the physical limitations of the body, instead experiencing the spiritual aspects of the Way while performing this form of moving meditation. Natural harmony, too, should be evident in the execution of all techniques as it applies to the human anatomy. By practicing within the constraints of the body's natural range of motion, stress and injury will be brought to a minimum. Likewise, permitting the muscles to remain in a relaxed and natural state will result in the development of explosive power upon impact. Consequently, since the Way is all encompassing in its relationship to physiology, natural movement equates to *do*. Clearly, from the early stages of social development on up to the present, an understanding of do has been accompanied by a deep appreciation of nature. In fact, one cannot exist without the other.

From this we began to see that Taoist philosophy has not only indirectly supplied the martial arts with a written agenda for concordant living, as portrayed in the *Tao Teh Ching* supported by its eighty-one separate advisories, but with a standard in the way of the Um/Yang to illustrate these beliefs. The *I Ching*, too, has contributed greatly in its illustration and recognition of the natural order of change as a precursor to an understanding of the Way. Furthermore, we can now identify ki and the duality of opposites as being two major principles that permeate traditional taekwondo philosophy. We would be remiss, then, if we did not acknowledge the great contribution Chinese culture has had on taekwondo in particular and the martial arts in general through Taoist doctrine. However, this should not be construed as an admission that taekwondo is devoid of its own genuine history. On the contrary, returning to a more native train of thought as it relates to the concept of do and the heritage of the Korean people, we travel back four thousand years to a period where the suggested progenitor of the Han race makes his appearance in the shape of the fabled Tan-gun.

It is said that in the days of Ko-Chosun, or ancient Korea, a divine being called Hwan-ung descended from heaven to the top of Mount T'ae-baek. Overhearing the prayers of a bear and tiger who greatly desired to take on human form, Hwan-ung offered to grant their wish under the condition that they remain secluded in a cave for a period of twenty-one days eating nothing but native herbs. Because of the tiger's innate restlessness, he was unable to meet these requirements. The bear, on the other hand, whose patience prevailed, exited the cave a beautiful maiden wanting nothing more than to have a child. Miraculously, following the transmission of Hwan-ung's breath of life, she gave birth to a son, naming him Tan-gun. Raised by the ancients, Tan-gun went on to help civilize the uncultivated tribes by teaching them farming, architecture, and various social graces. More importantly, however, the mythical founder is credited with the origination of traditional, national thought through his advocacy of *hongik-ingan* (the benefits of universal humanism) and *jaese-ihwa* (the rationalization of human living). These concepts, especially hongik-ingan which codifies the Korean sense of duty to the state, family and forbearers, constitute the foundation of a social framework that has blossomed into the uniquely Korean culture that exists today. Furthermore, the Han people needed to reconcile the ruthlessness of nature, the elements, and a highly restrictive lifestyle by clinging to a belief in the worship of "heaven's god" or impeccable virtuousness, later known as *seon*. According to the *Taekwon-do Textbook*, published under the auspices of the Kukkiwon, these doctrines have done much in contributing to the do or spirit of taekwondo as well as the overall character of traditional and contemporary Korean ethics.

Clearly, much in the way of traditional thought has gone into molding the modern concept of do in relationship to the martial arts. But, mythical perceptions notwithstanding, how do these ancient viewpoints merge with present philosophical thought in restoring what many today have lost in the way of ethical, spiritual, and physical direction? As we have seen from our research, a common thread that unites all martial arts is a belief in the fact that there is much more to gain from diligent training than the ability to kick higher or punch harder than the next person. Rather, by drawing on the experiences of those who have come before through written texts, traditional concepts, and approved technique, we develop a true sense of accomplishment, confidence, and self-esteem. Consequently, students of taekwondo often report stunning results after only a few short months of training as we can see from the following statements:"Even though I have been practicing for only three months, I am challenging my body, losing weight, learning self-defense along with a new language, and feeling good about myself again." "Since I have begun training, I have been thinking more about things around me. I am more compassionate and think more before I act." "Taekwondo has taught me balance both physically and spiritually." "Studying the martial art of taekwondo has created a strong foundation built on mind, body, and soul for me as well as my family."

Certainly, there are other vehicles that actively compete in supplying this essential emotional and physical gratification, but none are as comprehensive as the martial arts with its holistic approach. Where gymnastics or aerobics tend to fall short in their lack of philosophical depth and ritual commitment, traditional taekwondo and its sister disciplines succeed in satisfying these needs inasmuch as the simple repetition of movement results in enhanced health and a sense of well-being far beyond what can be obtained from the ordinary types of exercise. Likewise, religious or academic pursuits cannot be counted on to physically develop the body in the way determined practice can. Diligent training in taekwondo, on the other hand, coupled with a deep appreciation for the underlying philosophy it supports, provides one with a complete pallet of emotional, physical, and spiritual principles on which to model their life.

Furthermore, a vast majority of us tend to view change as a shock to the system, even though it is the one constant we can be virtually assured of. This is especially true as we age and become more set in our ways. Our work, family relationships, even our health often appear immune to change only to be disturbed at some point by the shifting sands of time. By conforming to a belief in the Um/Yang and the constant change it promotes, these disturbances may be buffered and more readily accepted with grace and maturity. Just as our ancestors were at first terrified by their lack of knowledge concerning astronomical events, accurate understanding brings with it a certain tranquility. Moreover, in today's complex society it has become the trend to gauge one's level of success and ultimate worth on material wealth rather than personal integrity and moral character. Since this is a recognized fact of life, the practitioner must be wary of the conflict this dilemma creates. But, while it is true that one needs a strong financial base in order to survive, it is important not to confuse the need for money and materialistic pursuits with the hope of happiness. Surely, the artificial comfort found in the elusive drive for financial security cannot match the satisfaction found in spiritual contentment, good health, and ethical behavior. By following the Way, however, the martial artist as citizen and provider is assured of a balanced life as expressed by the Um/Yang. This is accomplished through a sincere pursuit of the many virtues contained in the Way; these virtues are rooted in humility, compassion, courage, and wisdom.

The Way, then, is clearly paved by virtuous thought and action. It is arrived at through diligent practice and a never-ending commitment to excellence. To waver is an admission of one's humanity. To reclaim the rightful path, however, is a sure sign of discipline and valor. In the words of the Zen Buddhist patriarch, Bodhidharma: "All know the Way; few actually walk it." By this we can see that a courageous heart is needed in fostering a belief in non-conformity; that is, not falling prey to the excesses of a less dedicated, ethically deficient lifestyle. We discover, after a time, that the beneficial aspects of do begin to seep into every facet of daily living. Our sense of balance, both physically and spiritually, begins to increase. Better health ensues. Reflexes are sharpened and a profound appreciation for the value of life pervades our being. Finally, we are rewarded with greater confidence and self-respect through our knowledge of personal defense. Meanwhile, the course we have charted begins to unfold before us. This course is a journey marked by many milestones. It is a highway whose unbroken line leads to the physical, philosophical, and spiritual refinement of the individual. With each new revelation the practitioner comes closer to the ultimate goal of enlightenment. This journey, this road, is called taekwondo and it is defined by its simple ending, do. The Way or path of the martial artist is the road of hope and virtue we all must follow.

Warriors of a Different War

Triumphant in battle, you once again return to the Hwarang training grounds located high in the mountains overlooking the majestic expanse of the Kyongju plain. Here, you continue your studies in Eastern philosophy, music, poetry, weaponry, and kwonbop, the empty-hand fighting skill that will one day mature into the great Korean martial art of taekwondo. After the unification of the Three Kingdoms, comes a period of peace and prosperity for the Silla you fought so hard to preserve. Your gallant efforts have not gone unnoticed by your superiors, assuring you a position of respect and responsibility in a society based on community service born of national pride. And so, after long days locked in conflict, you sleep soundly safe in the knowledge that you have served your country with honor and virtue based on the strict code of honor you so fiercely embrace.

Although fictional in nature, the above scenario could easily parallel the life and times experienced by many of the young nobles selected to practice under the banner of Hwarang-do during the latter part of the seventh century. Historical fact does show us, however, that during the reign of united Silla's dynastic parties, a great many deeds and accomplishments were bestowed upon society at large. These cultural advances were in no small part influenced by the indomitable spirit and valor of the Hwarang. Accordingly, much of the financial, political, and cultural growth currently enjoyed by the Korean people can be directly attributed to the courage and virtuous behavior exemplified by these young warriors of the past. In visiting Korea, this connection becomes astonishingly clear and one cannot help but see the correlation between warrior-of-the-past and citizen-of-today, successfully battling under oddly familiar sets of circumstances. Even now it is evident that the spirit of the Hwarang pervades the collective consciousness of the Korean people in their quest for global parity.

But, with the wars of unification and the ghosts of the Hwarang relegated to history, fourteen centuries later, we are faced with yet a new set of challenges equally important to our own future development. Never before in the history of mankind has humanity been faced with so many complex and varied challenges. This has caused the average citizen to search far and wide for encouragement, wisdom, and leadership. However, rather than looking inward to the higher self for answers, the search has generally focused on external sources. Teachers are expected to act as surrogate parents. Structured religion dictates spiritual conformity. Meanwhile, one by one, humanity assumes the role of the victim. This trend will continue, unabashed, until individuals ultimately accept responsibility, not only for how their actions effects others, but for the actions that relate to their own personal success or failure in the world. The martial arts, with taekwondo leading the way, is one solution that offers a clear and concise path towards self-determination and enlightenment that will remedy many of the ills suffered by those seeking spiritual solace.

Consequently, with the worldwide proliferation of taekwondo, more and more people are becoming exposed to the virtues and benefits this great Korean martial art has to offer. Men, women, and children from all walks of life are becoming involved by taking a courageous first step towards self-fulfillment by crossing the threshold of a local dojang. Some cynics view this activity as merely a hollow trend that will go the way of other half-hearted philosophies driven by vogue and fashion. Others however, approach the martial arts with religious fervor. This behavior is not uncommon considering the inevitable catharsis that takes place in conjunction with diligent, sincere practice.

But how, one may ask, can a sport steeped in aggression, machismo and Eastern mysticism be expected to personify the essence of superior living? The answer is simple—if taekwondo provided only these principles, it could not further us along on our paths toward self-improvement. As we have discovered from our research, taekwondo is a ritualized, holistic discipline rich in tradition and aesthetic beauty with a strong ethical foundation etched from ancient philosophical ideologies. Because it is a true martial art tested in combat and not merely a sport, taekwondo contains a treasure trove of defensive techniques. Accordingly, the confidence it instills allows the practitioner to walk life's path unhindered by common fears, thus revealing simple wonders that always existed but were never before seen. Through an alliance with nature, the taekwondoist develops a true sense of his place in the universe and an appreciation for life in all its glory. Balance and moderation of temperament is achieved through an understanding of Eastern thought as expressed by that greatest of Taoist symbols, the Um/Yang.

Furthermore, since taekwondo is an action philosophy, the martial artist learns when to proceed and when to hesitate, never missing an opportunity but, by the same token, never acting hastily. Likewise, through a program of diligent practice, the student takes comfort in preparedness and his reaction will be measured and effective. Moreover, dedication to the martial arts breeds humility brought on by the realization that the practitioner is in possession of potentially lethal techniques that not only must be respected, but controlled. This humble demeanor is further characterized by the fact that taekwondo is not about any single individual. Rather, it is about a complex, scientifically rooted fighting art established centuries ago by a proud and noble people. Perhaps the single most important factor steering the martial artist in his quest for self-fulfillment is an adherence to a strict code of honor the principles of which have been handed down through the generations by warriors representing links in the great chain of knowledge.

In my own experience, there have been magic times when I have felt this inexorable bond with the past in a highly significant manner. One summer during a training excursion to Korea, I traveled to a remote village high in the southern mountains. After an intense session of meditation and a jog through the woods along a dirt path, our small group arrived at a clearing in the forest. We were enchanted by the breathtaking scenery surrounding us. Here, we were commanded by our instructors, Grand Master Cho and Master Jang, to assume a horse stance facing the mountains that towered above us not far in the distance. Our hosts spoke with reverence regarding the Hwarang warriors of the past and how they would draw power in prepara-

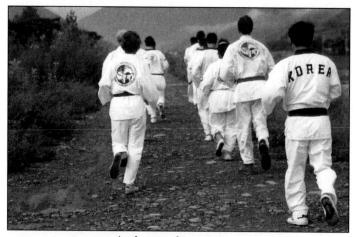

Jogging into the forests of Korea to train at sunrise.

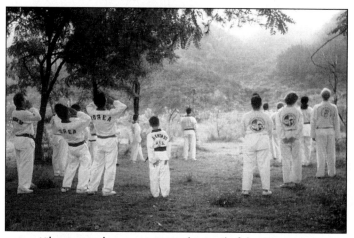

Kihoping at the mountains in the Land of the Hwarang.

tion for battle using the very method we were about to experience. Still in horse stance, we faced the majestic peaks and were directed to kihop as loud as possible. With our echoes reverberating off the rugged slopes, we absorbed the energy the mountains reflected back, and were told to share it with those in America. In that instant, I felt as if the spirits of the Hwarang had invaded my mind. Today, I am wondering if they ever left.

As martial artists we are warriors of a different war—a war against indifference, brutality, conformity, and fear. It is fought on a battlefield where the specter of complacency rules. Our defenses are many, wrought by the virtues a superior lifestyle demands. The armor we have chosen acts as protection against the fiery brands of jealousy, intimidation, and greed. Therefore, it is incumbent upon us as modern day warriors to continue in the tradition of the Hwarang—allowing courage to fill the void when confidence fails. We must set worthy examples for those around us and apply the virtues we have been taught in the hope of making a contribution, no matter how minor, in forging a better society. Because, ultimately, taekwondo is not a sport to be played within the confines of a set space and time. It is not a casual pastime, nor is it a garment to be taken on and off at will. Rather, taekwondo, in its traditional form, is a way of life.

The Training and Dynamic Meditation of Kyung Won University

Kyung Won University is located at 65 Bokjung-Dong in the Sujung-Gu district of Seoul, South Korea. It's sprawling campus contains all the modern facilities one would expect of a thriving academic institution. Classrooms, lecture halls, playing fields, gymnasiums and dormitories can be found within a short walk of one another. But, unlike its Western counterparts, Kyung Won offers a major in the native martial art of taekwon-do. Potential students apply from all over the country in the hope of gaining admittance to what is perhaps the most intense martial arts training program in the world. A chosen few who endure will undoubtedly go on to become members of the elite Korean national taekwondo team eventually representing their country as Olympic athletes.

On the top floor of a building situated in the center of the complex is the University's training hall or dojang. As we climbed the circular flight of concrete steps leading to the

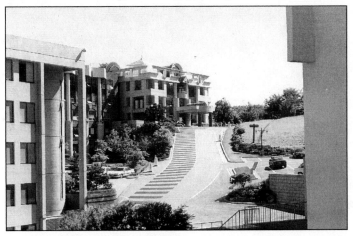

Kyung Won University.

entrance, I realized that over five-thousand miles and nearly two days journey separated us from our home and this much-anticipated point in time.

Korea was no stranger to me. I had visited "the land of the morning calm" some years before, training and traveling in what amounted to be the most enlightening experience of my life as a martial artist thus far. I had promised myself that someday I, too, would offer my own students an opportunity to share in a similar experience. However, this trip promised to be even more enriching since we would be traveling in the company of Grand Master Richard Chun, 9th degree black belt, director of the Richard Chun Taekwondo Center in New York City and president of the United States Taekwondo Association. Because of Grand Master Chun's presence, doors, normally closed, would open wide permitting a view of taekwondo that is often hidden from the eyes of Westerners.

As we entered the dojang I noticed that a large stage dominated a training area measuring roughly fifty by one hundred feet, all told. Kicking targets, heavy bags, head gear and chest protectors or hogu, littered the perimeter. The natural light streaming in through the tall windows that peaked at the arched ceiling, amplified the contrasting colors of the orange and green puzzle mat. A banner beckoning us to embrace "the Dream of Taekwon" hung above the entry way.

Expectations high, we crowded into a tiny locker room, replaced our clothes with the traditional V-neck uniform or dobok worn by the taekwondo practitioner, and quickly entered the gymnasium. Grand Master Chun, along with our host for the day, Professor Kyu Seok Lee, had been seated in a row of chairs on the raised platform offering them a unique vantage point from which to view our training. As we were called to attention in strict militaristic fashion by Professor Lee's head instructor, Master Jang Ki Park, a solidly built tactician, amicable yet demanding of respect, it became apparent that our numbers had grown significantly. A contingent of Kyung Won students, in conjunction with members of the Syrian national team, were on hand to mutually participate in the advanced training program. Bows of respect were exchanged and Professor Lee rose to deliver a brief lecture underlining the importance of focus and perseverance. Grand Master Chun, being well known throughout the world taekwondo community, reciprocated with inspirational words of encouragement. Finally, after months of wonder, our first day of training in Korea, the homeland of taekwondo, was about to begin. In retrospect, we were not disappointed. The training that followed was extremely difficult and required great stamina. But, since we were acclimated to practicing in this manner back home, it did not overwhelm us. Our group was composed of a mixed ranking of students ranging in age from ten to fifty years old. At no point during our seven day stay did anyone complain or abstain from training.

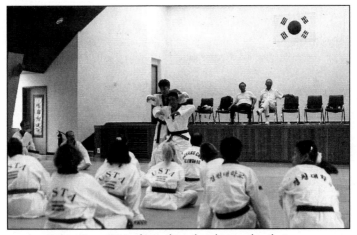

Master Jang Ki Park teaching ho shin sool techniques.

As a prelude to our practice we began with a set of exercises intended to condition the muscles and heat the body's core. These consisted of jumping jacks, sit-ups, push-ups and static stretches followed by a series of relays similar in nature to those I had been exposed to at the Korean National University for Physical Education during my prior excursion. Mindful of building team spirit, we ran, jumped, evaded and crawled in six lines of ten students each, from one side of the dojang to the other. Prepared now for an increase in intensity, the kicking drills began in earnest. Kwung Won students, sporting the University's logo on the back of their doboks, stood at the head of each line holding a kicking target. One by one we executed round, hook, spinning hook, jumping round, back and push kicks to the targets in an effort to enhance our technique.

An hour later we began perfecting our poom-se or forms. These are formal exercises aimed at defeating multiple, imaginary attackers coming from different directions. Since Kyung Won adheres to the rules and regulations of the Korea Taekwondo Association and the World Taekwondo Federation, color belts practiced the Taegeuk forms while the various degree black belts performed Koryo, Keumgang and Taebaek.

Thoroughly exhausted, it was time for lunch at the University's cafeteria. Professor Lee and his associates treated us to a generous repast of sliced marinated beef over rice complimented by kimchee, the ubiquitous pickled cabbage served at every meal. In an attempt to regain our strength we rested for awhile, lounging beneath the pavilions and and ginkgo trees of the campus.

At the invitation of Professor Kyu Seok Lee, we joined him in his classroom. Chalk in hand, he spoke of the influence the three major Asian philosophies of Buddhism, Taoism and Confucianism exerted on taekwondo. Master Lee had trained many champions during his tenure at Kyung Won. He looked to be in his fifties with short black hair and a trim body that housed a stern demeanor. At the close of his seminar, the Professor gifted me with a copy of a book he had authored entitled: *A Guide to Taekwondo...History, Philosophy & Training Methods.*

At the resumption of our training, Master Park, possibly sensing the effect the hot afternoon was having on his students, began with a remarkable method of dynamic meditation. Seated in a half-lotus position we performed a deep breathing exercise coupled with a series of arm stretches and body-bends that seemed instantly to reignite our internal ki energy. Much refreshed, we were now prepared for the rigorous self-defense and sparring drills that lay ahead. With the help of Master Sang Bum Yoon, Jang Ki Park demonstrated a number of effective ho shin sool or self-defense tactics, intended to disarm, disable or subdue an attacker. Master Yoon was a cheerful, young martial artist who spoke fluent English and was quick to smile. Aside from managing the taekwondo program at Yong In University, another of Korea's premiere martial arts schools, Mr. Yoon was a graduate of the Hwarang Educational Institute, and our instructor, liaison and traveling companion for the entire trip. It was gratifying to see that the traditional aspects of taekwondo, those of a purely defensive nature, were not dismissed by the attending masters in favor of the sportive elements so prevalent in the martial arts today.

In preparation for WTF style, full-contact sparring, a training feature many in our group found most desirable, Professor Lee with one of his most able students in tow, demonstrated the "twenty-five second drill". In this drill person A, who is the holder, rotates a kicking target through the four compass points causing student B, the defender, to circulate within each quadrant while executing a combination of kicking techniques. Anyone attempting this drill for the first time, aside from realizing the value of aerobic conditioning, quickly comes to appreciate the dual roles agility and focus play in taekwondo.

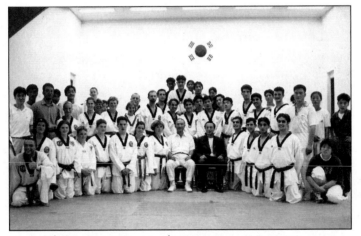

The Korean, Syrian, and USTA Teams at Kyung Won.

At this point, those wishing to participate were directed to don fighting gear and prepare to face fellow martial artists who had traveled thousands of miles to benefit from the cooperative effort inherent in team practice. Admittedly, it is one thing to spar with students within one's own school and another altogether to go eye to eye with a practitioner from around the world. However, this is precisely why many of our students elected to visit Korea in the first place: to develop courage in the face of danger while cultivating martial arts skill in harmony with others. It was remarkable to observe the ensuing matches. Each taekwondoist favored, as one would expect, a particular technique, executing it is superb fashion. One of the most notable characteristics of the Korean practitioners was the blinding speed with which they delivered blow after blow. This was international competition practice at its finest with the Korean team facing the Syrian team and, subsequently, or USTA team facing both.

Throughout our training at Kyung Won University the five tenets of taekwondo were in evidence. Courtesy, integrity, perseverance, self-control and indomitable spirit were not only the rule of the day, but essential components of the overall program. Our group went on from Kyung Won to visit the famed Kukkiwon, headquarters to taekwondo worldwide, the Korean National University for Physical Education, the Kouk Sun-Do School of ki development and Bulguksa Temple, one of the greatest monuments to Buddhism in Asia.

These are merely some of the highlights of our visit to Kyung Won University and our journey to "The Land of the Morning Calm". Driving through the countryside, one cannot help but admire the lush, terraced farm lands and rich, rolling hills. Korea's cities meanwhile, are at the same time both modern and rustic in many ways. With much new construction taking place the streets are as clogged with traffic as they are in any major Western city. But, perhaps most importantly, by visiting the elegant temples, shrines and academic institutions dedicated to the birth and development of the martial arts, one not only begins to feel a physical connection to taekwondo, but a geographical and chronological connection as well. Clearly, this is a pilgrimage every taekwondoist should aspire to make at some point during their practice of the Korean martial arts.

Dynamic Meditation

*as taught to the author by Master Jang Ki Park,
Professor, Department of Taekwondo, Kyung Won
University*

Kyung Won students view dynamic meditation as a bridge
between seated meditation intended to clear the mind and the
formal warm-up routine. It serves to prepare the musculature for
both static and dynamic flexibility exercises while reigniting ki
(internal energy) through deep breathing. Each posture should
be clocked to the duration of a normal inhalation and an exhalation with a two second pause between motions. One cycle normally takes one minute to complete.

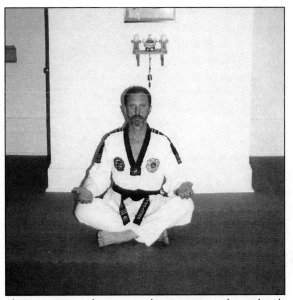

Photo #1: Begin the exercise by sitting cross-legged with
the hands on the knees palms up.

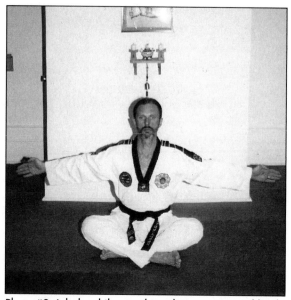

Photo #2: Inhale while stretching the arms out and back.

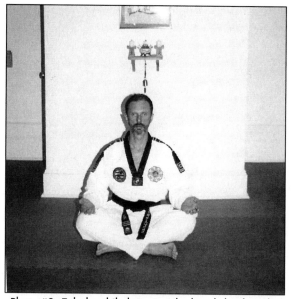

Photo #3: Exhale while bringing the hands back to the
starting position.

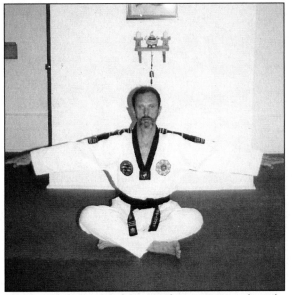

Photo #4: Inhale while bringing the arms out to the side palms down.

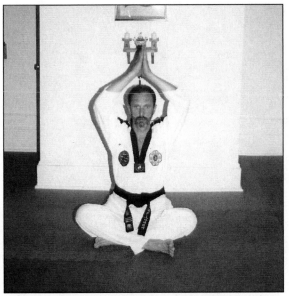

Photo #5: Exhale while raising the hands above the head palms touching and then inhale.

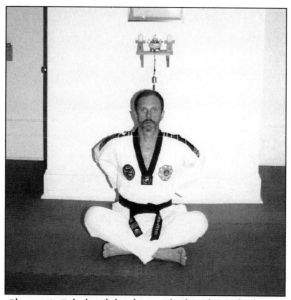

Photo #6: Exhale while placing the hands on the lower back palms over kidneys.

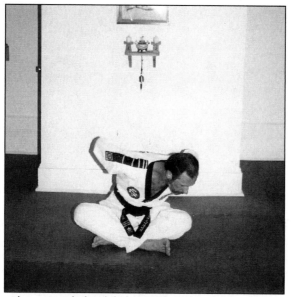

Photo #7: Inhale while bringing the head down to the left knee.

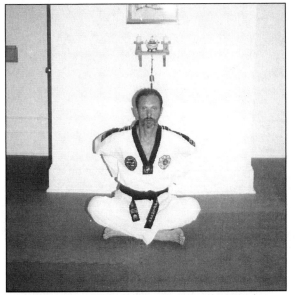

Photo #8: Exhale while returning to the upright position.

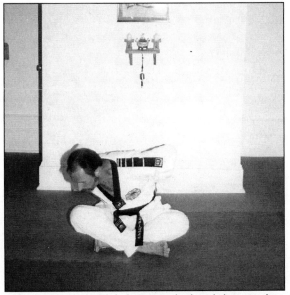

Photo #9: Inhale while bringing the head down to the right knee.

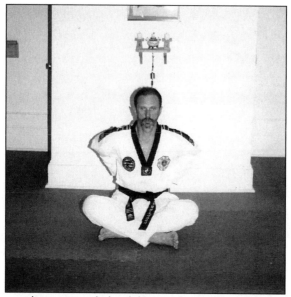

Photo #10: Exhale while returning to the upright position.

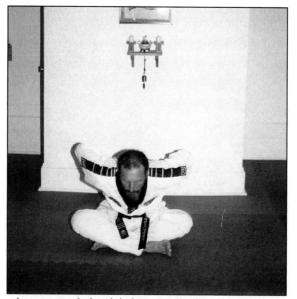

Photo #11: Inhale while bringing the head down to the center.

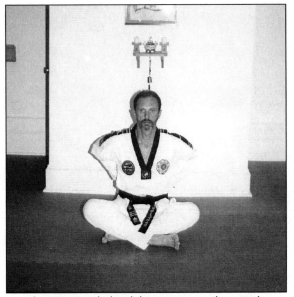

Photo #12: Exhale while returning to the upright position.

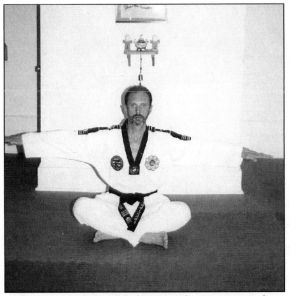

Photo #13: Inhale while bringing the arms out to the side palms down.

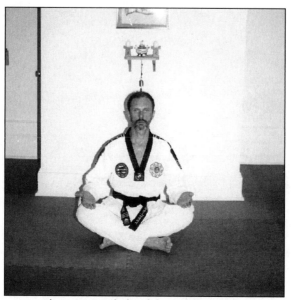

Photo #14: Exhale while returning to the
starting position.

Martial Arts Organizations

Amateur Athletic Union (AAU)
    1910 Hotel Plaza Blvd., Lake Buena Vista, FL 32830, USA
    (407) 934-7200 www.aausports.org

International Hapkido Federation (IHF)
    3201 Santa Monica Boulevard, Santa Monica, CA 90404,
    USA
    (310) 829-2643 www.intl-hapkido.org

International Taekwondo Federation (ITF)
    Drau Gasse 3, A-1210 Vienna, Austria
    (43-1) 292-8467 www.itf-taekwondo.com

Korea National Tourism Organization (KNTO)
    Two Executive Drive, Fort Lee, NJ 07024, USA
    (201) 585-0909 www.knto-th.org

Korea Taekwondo Association (KTA)
    Olympic Park 88-2 Oryun-dong, Songpa-gu, Seoul, Korea
    (02) 420-4271 www.koreataekwondo.org

The Kukkiwon (World Taekwondo Headquarters)
    Yuk Sam-dong, Kang Nam-ku, Seoul, 135-080, Korea
    567-3204, 1058

The Richard Chun Taekwondo Center
    220 East 86th Street, New York, NY 10028, USA
    (212) 772-8918 www.chunmartialarts.com

United States Taekwondo Association (USTA)
    220 East 86th Street, New York, NY 10028, USA
    (212) 772-8918 www.ustkda.com

United States Taekwondo Union (USTU)
    One Olympic Park Place, Suite 405, Colorado Springs, CO
    80909, USA
    (719) 578-4632 www.ustu.org

World Taekwondo Federation (WTF)
    635 Yuksamdong, Kangnamku, Seoul 135-080, Korea
    82-2-566-2505 www.worldsport.com

Yang's Martial Arts Association (YMAA)
    4354 Washington Street, Boston, MA 02131, USA
    (617) 323-7215 www.ymaa.com

To Contact the Author
Chosun Taekwondo Academy
    P.O. Box 721, Warwick, NY 10990, USA
    (845) 986-2288 www.chosuntkd.com

Korean/English Translations for Taekwondo Terms and Techniques

Stances

Ap Koobi	Front stance
Dwi Koobi	Back stance
Ja Choom Sogi	Horse stance
Ap Sogi	Walking stance
Kyorugi Jase	Fighting stance
Bom Sogi	Cat stance
Koa Sogi	Cross stance
Hakdari Sogi	Crane stance

Kicking Techniques

Ap Chagi	Front kick
Dollyo Chagi	Roundhouse kick
Yop Chagi	Side kick
Dwi Chagi	Back kick
Naeryo Chagi	Ax kick
Pyojok Chagi	Crescent kick
Miro Chagi	Push kick
Momdollyo	
Dwidolloyo Chagi	Turning hook kick
Hurio Chagi	Wheel kick
Twio Chagi	Jumping kick
Goollo Chagi	Hop kick
Bandal Chagi	Half Moon kick
Nalla Chagi	Flying kick
Opo Chagi	Falling kick
Doobal	
Dangsang Chagi	Double jumping kicks

Punching Techniques

Momtong Jiluki	Middle punch
Olgool Jiluki	High punch
Alle Jiluki	Low punch
Bandae Jiluki	Reverse punch
Baro Jiluki	Lunge punch
Chi Jiluki	Uppercut punch
Yop Jiluki	Side punch
Dollyo Jiluki	Round punch
Sewo Jiluki	Vertical punch
Koondol Joki	Hook punch

Dikootja Jiluki	C punch
Doo Chumok Jiluki	Double punch

Striking Techniques

Me Chumok	Hammer fist
Doong Chumok	Back fist
Bam Chumok	Middle finger fist
Pyun Chumok	Flat fist
Batang Sohn Chilki	Palm heel strike
Sohnnal Chilki	Knife hand strike
Sohnnal	
Sohnnal Doong Chilki	Ridge hand strike
Pyun Sohnkoot Chilki	Spear hand strike
Kawi Sohnkoot Chilki	Two finger strike
Inji Shonkoot Chilki	Single finger strike
Akum Sohn Chilki	Tiger mouth strike
Gom Sohn Chilki	Bear hand strike
Sohn Doong Chilki	Back hand strike
Sohn Mok Chilki	Ox Jaw strike
Palkup Chilki	Elbow strike
Moorup Chilki	Knee strike
Mohri Chilki	Head strike

Blocking Techniques

Alle Makki	Low block
Olgool Makki	High block
Ahn Momtong Makki	Out/In middle block
Bakat Momtong Makki	In/Out middle block
Ahn Han Sohnnal Makki	Out/In single knife hand block
Bakat Han Sohnnal Makki	In/Out single knife hand block
Dool Sohnnal Momtong Makki	Double knife hand block
Ghodulo Makki	Double closed first block
Otkolo Makki	X block
Gawi Makki	Scissors block
Hecho Makki	Spread block
Yop Makki	Side block
Batang Sohn Makki	Palm heel block
Sohn Mok Makki	Wrist block
Sohnnal Doong Makki	Ridge hand block
Sohn Doong Makki	Back hand block
Pyojok Chagi Makki	Crescent kick block

Basic Terminology

Cha Riot	Attention
Joombi	Ready
Kyung Ye	Bow
Bal Pak Ko	Switch stance
Dwi Ro Dora	About face
Si Jak	Begin
Barro	Return to ready
Goo Man	End
Kibon	Basics
Kibon Dong Chak	Basic movements
Makki	Block
Jiluki	Punch
Chilki	Strike
Chagi	Kick
Poom Se	Traditional choreographed forms
Il Su Shik	One-step sparring
Ho Shin Sool	Self-defense techniques
Kyuk Pa	Breaking
Kyorugi	Sparring
Kwan Jang Nim	Grand Master
Sa Bum Nim	Master
Kyo Sa Nim	Instructor
Sun Ba Nim	Senior
Dojang	Training hall
Dobok	Uniform
Ti	Belt
Kukki	Flag
Muk Yum	Meditation
Soom Sha Ki	Deep breathing
Wen	Left
Ohren	Right

Counting

Hana	One
Dool	Two
Set	Three
Net	Four
Dasoot	Five
Yasoot	Six
Il Gop	Seven
Yodol	Eight
Ahop	Nine
Yol	Ten

Glossary

Aikido: The "Way of Harmonizing Energy." A Japanese system of locks and throws centered on using an opponent's negative energy against him. Founded by Morihei Ueshiba, also known as "O-Sensei."

Beginner's Mind: A principle of Zen Buddhism supporting an innocent and open outlook on practice.

Bodhidharma: Zen patriarch thought to be the founder of Chinese Shaolin gongfu.

Bokken: A wooden sword used in the practice of Kumdo and Kendo.

Buddhism: An Eastern philosophy turned religion focusing on self-purification and meditation. Founded by Siddhartha Gautama.

Bojutsu: The Japanese art of staff fighting.

Bushido: The samurai code of honor. The "way of the warrior."

Chung Do Kwan: The "School of the True Path." One of the original Korean martial art schools founded by Won Kuk Lee in 1944.

Confucianism: An Eastern philosophy based on social values and the role of the "superior man." Founded by the Chinese philosopher, Confucius.

Cosmic Mudra: A traditional hand gesture shaped by placing the back of one hand in the palm of the other while allowing the tips of the thumbs to touch.

Dan: A grade of black belt ranging from one to ten.

Do: The "Way" or "Path" to enlightenment. The philosophical component of a martial art.

Dobok: The v-neck uniform worn by a practitioner of taekwondo.

Dojang: A designated place where one comes to study the "Way." A school where Korean martial arts are taught.

Gi: The traditional wrap-around uniform generally worn by practitioners of the Japanese martial arts.

Gongfu: Literally translated as "good effort." A generic term for many forms of Chinese martial arts. (Also spelled "kung fu.)

Gup: A grade given to the color belt taekwondo practitioner before the attainment of the black belt.

Hapkido: The "Way of Harmony." A Korean martial art focusing on throws, locks, hand strikes, and kicks. Rich in defensive value and the cultivation of ki.

Hogu: A chest protector used during sparring practice.

Ho Shin Sool: A Korean term for self-defense techniques.

Holistic Approach: The principle of martial arts practice that advocates uniting the mind, body, and spirit.

Hwarang: An elite group of young Sillian warriors schooled in philosophy, ethics, and native martial arts.

Hwarang-do: The "Way of Flowering Manhood." A set of ethical principles followed by the warriors of the Hwarang.

Hyung: A form or set of offensive and defensive techniques performed in sequence. (See: Poom-se, Kata)

I Ching: The ancient *Chinese Book of Changes.* Used as an oracle for guidance or forecasting future events.

ITF: The International Taekwondo Federation. Currently under the direction of General Choi Hong Hi.

Il Su Shik: A traditional Korean term for one-step sparring. A prearranged drill where one partner advances one step with an attack while the other defends.

In/Yo: A Japanese term for the "duality of opposites." (See: Yin/Yang, Um/Yang.)

Jeet Kune Do: The "Way of the Intercepting Fist." A fighting style founded by martial artist and movie star Bruce Lee.

Judo: The "Compliant Way." A Japanese martial art and sport centering on turning an opponent's aggression against him. Founded by Jigoro Kano in 1882.

Jook Do: A Korean term for the bamboo sword.

Jung Bong: A Korean term for the fighting staff. Known as a "Bo" in Japanese.

Karate: Literally translated as "empty hand." An Okinawan and Japanese martial art practiced in many iterations. Thought to be founded on fighting principles originating in China.

Kata: A pattern of offensive and defensive techniques practiced in a predetermined sequence by the student of the Japanese martial arts.

Katana: The sword used by the samurai warrior.

Kendo: A Japanese martial art translated as the "Way of the Sword."

Kenjutsu: A Japanese martial art that stresses the practical use of the sword.

Ki: Korean and Japanese expression for the internal life force used by martial artists to amplify technique.

Kihop: The vocal manifestation of the internal life force uttered by the martial artist to increase focus and power. Called "Kiai" in Japanese.

Koan: An illogical poem meant to overwhelm the mind while in search of satori.

Kobukson: A Korean battleship dubbed the "Turtle Boat." It was invented by Admiral Yi, Sun-sin in the 1500's and is thought to be the predecessor of the modern submarine.

Kong Soo Do: "Empty Hands Way." An early name given to the Korean martial art that eventually evolved into taekwondo.

Kukkiwon: The "National Gymnasium" located in Seoul, Korea. Home of the WTF and the center of taekwondo operations worldwide.

Kumdo: An ancient martial art and system of native Korean sword fighting.

Kwan: School or gymnasium. One of the original Korean martial arts schools.

Kyuk Pa: Korean term for breaking techniques.

Laogong: An area at the center of the palm thought to be sensitive to ki energy.

Mantra: A phrase or word repeated during the process of meditation as a way of focusing and centering the individual.

Meditation: A method of freeing or quieting the mind while in a seated, formal posture. Also used for visualization and relaxation.

Moo Duk Kwan: The "School of Martial Virtue." One of the original Korean martial art schools founded by Hwang Kee in 1945.

Mudra: A hand gesture used during the practice of meditation. Also used to seal in ki energy.

Muk Yum: A Korean term for meditation.

Muyedobo-Tongji: The "Illustrated Manual of Martial Arts" published in the 1790's. A Korean scholarly work depicting native martial art techniques.

Mushin: The Zen concept of mind/no mind.

Oh Do Kwan: The "School of My Way." One of the original Korean martial art schools founded by General Choi Hong Hi in 1953.

Palgwe: A set of eight traditional Korean taekwondo poom-se emphasizing low stances.

Poom-Se: A choreographed sequence of taekwondo techniques aimed at defeating imaginary opponents attacking from various directions. (See: Kata, Hyung)

Presence of Mind: The ability to remain calm and analytical in stressful situations.

Qi: The internal life force, as expressed in Chinese, used by martial artists to amplify technique. (Also see: Ki).

Qigong: An ancient Chinese healing art with martial overtones based on the manipulation and balancing of chi.

Satori: The Zen term for sudden enlightenment.

Sesok Ogye: The "Code of the Hwarang." Five ethical commandments handed down by the Buddhist monk Wonkwang Popsa.

Shinai: A bamboo sword used in the practice of Kumdo and Kendo.

Shintoism: A Japanese religion characterized by devotion to natural deities and a belief that the Emperor is a direct descendant of the Sun Goddess.

Shin Shin Totsu Aikido: "Aikido with Mind and Body Coordinated." A form of aikido founded by Koichi Tohei.

Shaolin Temple: The legendary seat of Chinese martial arts located in Hunan province, China.

Sieza: A formal kneeling posture used during meditation practice.

Song Jul Kwan: The nunchaku. A weapon constructed of two short baton-like objects connected by a length of chain or rope.

Soo Bahk Do: The "Way of Striking Hand." A Korean martial art established by Kwang Kee upon his return to Korea from China.

Student Creed: A group of tenets or moral principles recited by martial artists during the closing ritual of a class.

Subahk: An ancient Korean martial art dating back to the Koguryo dynasty.

Tae Soo Do: "Kick Fist Way." An early name given to the Korean martial art that would eventually evolve into taekwondo.

Taegeuk: A set of eight modern taekwondo poom-se emphasizing upright fighting stances.

Taekkyon: A native Korean martial art emphasizing circular kicking techniques.

Taekwondo: The "Way of Smashing with Hands and Feet." A Korean martial art drawn from traditional taekkyon and subahk, but based on the circular principles of Chinese gongfu coupled with the linear strikes of Japanese karate.

Taijiquan (Tai Chi Chuan): The "Grand Ultimate Fist." An internal Chinese martial art influenced by the principles of the I Ching. Practiced primarily to promote health.

Tan Tien: A Chinese expression for the energy center located two inches below the navel where the internal life force resides.

Tang Soo Do: The "Way of the China Hand." A Korean martial art with similarities to shotokan karate. Founded by Hwang Kee in 1949.

Tao: Chinese expression for the "Way" or "Path." The universal governing force of nature as put forth in Lao Tzu's *Tao Teh Ching.*

Tao Teh Ching: The "Way of Virtue." The collected works of Lao Tzu written during the fourth century B.C. The centerpiece of Taoist tradition.

Taoism: A Chinese philosophy based on the concept of non-intervention and conformity to the Tao. Founded on the teachings of Lao Tzu.

Telegraphing: Wrongly demonstrating one's intentions to an opponent during sparring.

Third Eye: An area at the center of the forehead thought to be sensitive to ki.

Tjan Tjin: A Korean expression for the energy center located two inches below the navel where the internal life force resides. (See: Tan Tien.)

Tjan Tjin Ho Hup: Deep breathing exercises practiced during meditation aimed at cultivating internal ki energy.

Um/Yang: Korean symbol expressing harmony between opposites. (See: Yin/Yang, In/Yo.)

USTA: The United States Taekwondo Association. Currently under the direction of Grand Master Richard Chun.

USTU: The United States Taekwondo Union. This is the national governing body for sport taekwondo in America.

Warrior Way: A set of ethical principles the martial artist lives by.

WTF: The World Taekwondo Federation. Currently under the direction of Dr. Un Yong Kim.

Wushu: A group of modern Chinese martial arts practiced primarily for their entertainment and competitive value.

Yin/Yang: An ancient Taoist symbol expressing harmony between opposites. (See: Um/Yang, In/Yo.)

Yudo: A Korean derivative of Japanese judo.

Zazen: A form of seated Zen meditation.

Zen: An Eastern philosophy and Buddhist sect based on the realization of enlightenment through meditation.

Bibliography

Chun, Rhin Moon Richard. *Taekwondo: A Korean Martial Art.*
New York: Harper & Row, 1976.

Chun, Rhin Moon Richard. *Advancing in Taekwondo.*
New York: Harper & Row, 1983.

Deshimaru, Taisen. *Zen Way to the Martial Arts.*
New York: Penguin Books, 1982.

Kauz, Herman. *The Martial Spirit.*
New York: Overlook Press, 1977.

Kim, Daeshik. *Taekwondo.*
Korea: NANAM Publishing Co., 1991.

Kim, Un Yong. *The Taekwon-do Textbook.*
Korea: Oh Sung Publishers, 1995.

LeShan, Lawrence. *How to Meditate.*
New York: Bantam Books, 1974.

Mitchell, Richard L. *The History of Taekwondo Patterns.*
Lilley Gulch Taekwondo, 1987.

Morgan, Forrest E. *Living the Martial Way.*
New Jersey: Barricade Books, 1992.

Park Yeon Hee, Park Yeon Hwan, Gerrard, Jon., *Taekwondo: The
Ultimate Guide to the Word's Most Popular Martial Art.*
New York: *Facts on File, Inc.,* 1986.

Reed, William. *Ki: A Practical Guide for Westerners.*
Japan: Japan Publications, 1986.

Shim, Sang Kyu. *Promise and Fulfillment in the Art of Taekwondo.*
Iowa: TKD Enterprises, 1974.

Shim, Sang Kyu. *The Making of a Martial Artist.*
Iowa: TKD Enterprises, 1980.

Suzuki, Shunryu. *Zen Mind, Beginner's Mind.*
New York: Weatherhill Inc., 1970.

Tohei, Koichi. *Ki In Daily Life.*
Japan: Ki No Kenkyukai Headquarters, 1978.

Wei, Wu. *I-Ching Life: Living It.*
California: Power Press, 1996.

Yang, Jwing Ming. *Qigong for Health and Martial Arts.*
Massachusetts: YMAA, 1985.

About the Author

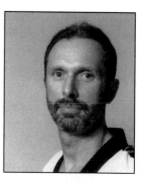

Doug Cook holds a third degree black belt in the Korean martial art of taekwondo, and is certified as an instructor by the United States Taekwondo Association and World Taekwondo Federation. After training twice in Korea, he went on to become a five-time gold medalist in the New York State Championships and the New York State Governor's cup competitions. He holds a D3 status as a U.S. referee and has received high honors from Korea in the form of a "Letter of Appreciation" presented by Grand Master Richard Chun, and signed by World Taekwondo Federation president, Dr. Un Yong Kim.

The author and his students are credited with the creation of the Chosun Women's Self-Defense Course—an effective workshop geared towards women of all ages, generally offered to corporate or civic groups as a community service. Recently, in response to a request for training from the U.S. Army National Guard/42nd Division, the author developed the Chosun Military Self-Defense course.

The author is a self-described traditionalist and places great emphasis on the underlying philosophical principles surrounding taekwondo. He demonstrates this belief by infusing meditation, breathing exercises, strong basic skills, and attention to the classic forms in his instruction.

Aside from continuing his martial arts education in New York City under the tutelage of world-renowned, ninth degree black belt, Grand Master Richard Chun, the author owns and operates the Chosun Taekwondo Academy located in Warwick, New York. The academy specializes in traditional instruction and internal energy development.

The author currently shares his knowledge of taekwondo through a series of articles he has written for *Black Belt* and other martial arts magazines. He is editor of the *United States Taekwondo Association Journal.*

Index

BOOKS FROM YMAA

more products available from...

YMAA Publication Center, Inc. 楊氏東方文化出版中心

1-800-669-8892 • ymaa@aol.com • www.ymaa.com

VIDEOS FROM YMAA

DVDS FROM YMAA

more products available from...
YMAA Publication Center, Inc. 楊氏東方文化出版中心

1-800-669-8892 • ymaa@aol.com • www.ymaa.com